"I recently had to speak in public. It was sprung as a surprise on me. At first I panicked. Then I reminded myself "you are an Ironman". Whenever I am scared, I picture the mass swim start, and remind myself that if I can do that, I can do anything."

-   **Bianca from South Africa, IRONMAN Switzerland finisher**

A challenge is only a challenge until you achieve it!
Good luck, Tiffany

1

IRONWOMEN

by
Tiffany Jolowicz

Iron wish, iron will, Ironwomen.

An inspiring insight into how and why women do
long distance triathlons.

This book is dedicated to my siblings, love you both.

I would like to thank my husband, Roland who has always been there to support me in this crazy triathlon mission. He has flown intercontinentally for weekends in order to be cheering along the course and at the finish line. He has listened to my training woes and successes. He has offered constructive and insightful advice, fully aware of how tactfully these had to be delivered. He combed through this book laboriously, spotting inconsistencies and run-on sentences. He has taken most of the photos, including the cover photo, which I think is a work of art. He ferries me to events at the crack of dawn and looks after the kids when I am off training. He brings me a cup of coffee early before I go off for a run and he leans down and gives me a congratulatory kiss at the end of each race. In short, without him I would not be an ironwoman and this book would never have happened. He is perfect and I love him, thank you for everything, Roland.

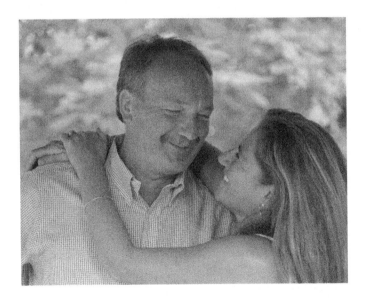

PART 1 – MY JOURNEY

SECTION1: AARHUS HALF TRIATHLON 2011

SECTION 2: BUITRAGO HALF TRIATHLON 2012

SECTION 3: IRONMAN SWITZERLAND 2013

SECTION 4: CHALLENGE ROTH ULTRA DISTANCE TRI 2015

PART 2 - MY 40 TRI-SISTERS' JOURNEY

In compliance with the World Triathlon Corporation guidelines for referencing brands, the generic term "full," or "ultra" distance will be used to describe the 226 km (3.8 km swim, 180 km bike & 42.2 km run) triathlon event and the term "half distance" will be used to describe the 70,3 km (1.9 km swim, 90 km bike & 21.1 km run) triathlon event. IRONMAN refers specifically to an event run by the World Triathlon Corporation

This book is jam packed with fun stories and lots of tips. It is not intended as a training programme for a long distance triathlon. Before starting on a vigorous exercise programme please see your doctor

Introduction:

IRONMAN Switzerland, Zürich, 28 July 2013,10 pm.

I completed the last kilometre in 4 minutes and 40 seconds, the fastest kilometre I have ever run in any of my 12 marathons and 30-odd half-marathons. I turned the corner, ran under the big red arch we had passed at 6.50am that morning and entered the final corridor. It was so over-powering that I did not even hear the announcement, "Tiffany Jolowicz you.are.an.IRONMAN." I crossed the finish line, my kids running with me. Roland, my husband, gave me a big kiss and my family, my fellow Zürich-Ironman finishers and friends, Kirsten and Maria and their families surrounded me. It was unbelievable. I was shaking all over. Tears ran down my face. A volunteer fought through the bodies to give me my medal, my IRONMAN medal! 15 hours and 2 minutes. Riding the heady mixture of physical exhaustion and mental over-charge, I went in search of my Ironman Switzerland T-shirt. Looking at the other women's lean faces in the finish tent, I sensed an energy, a powerful strength, a deep confidence in their eyes. Strangers but sisters, we hugged and offered congratulations and tears welled up in my eyes once more. We understood without saying a word what had happened out there today. That evening in Zürich, I realised that every woman who had completed IRONMAN Switzerland would have a tale to tell. I felt compelled to share this raw energy and sense of empowerment with other women. I wrote to IRONMAN Switzerland asking if they would permit me to send a questionnaire to all the female participants, they agreed. The idea for an ultra distance triathlon book about women, by women, for women was born. IRONWOMEN is the tales from my tri-sisters interwoven around mine. Together we share a wealth of knowledge, experience, insights, along with entertaining and inspiring stories. The Zürich athletes recount their fears and their failures, how they juggled commitments and relished their strengths and successes. This is our story, how and why we women took on the full distance triathlon challenge. All of this cumulative information will help any woman on a quest to take on a great challenge, or maybe, to finish a triathlon, no matter what the distance. I hope our stories inspire you. Kirsten, Maria and I had trained for two and a half years for Ironman Zürich. We started with hardly any knowledge. Together we set, broke down and pushed boundaries. We pooled our iron wish and became Ironwomen. We hadn't relied on a trainer and we never belonged to a Triathlon club. We jumped into the challenge and learned along the way. I documented our journey. This book is written for any woman who is aspiring to take on any distance triathlon and is looking for friends who have already done it.

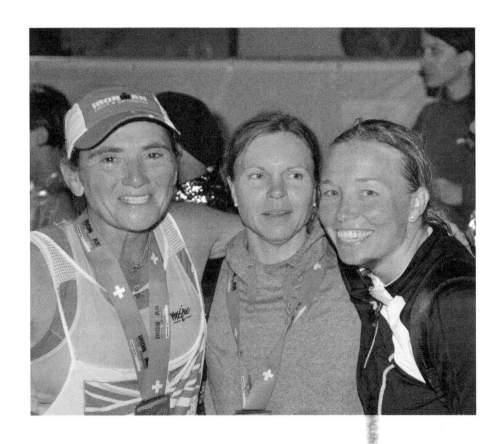

Tiffany   Maria   Kirsten

Ironman Switzerland was a fantastic journey, which also brought the gift of a friendship I cherish. I look forward to more adventures with Kirsten and Maria together as our hair goes grey and our legs stiffen. We will always be safe in the knowledge, that no one can take away our iron will.

Part I
MY JOURNEY

The urge to run IRONMAN Switzerland did not come out of the blue; it was born over time. My running career started in Duluth, Minnesota, USA in 1993, at age 28, when I half-walked, half-ran a half marathon in 2 hours and 43 minutes. 22 years later, July 2015, at age 50, I finished my second ultra distance triathlon, Challenge Roth in Germany.

The highlights of my triathlon career have been 4 events:

1) AARHUS HALF DISTANCE TRIATHLON, 2011
2) BUITRAGO HALF-DISTANCE TRIATHLON, 2012,
3) IRONMAN SWITZERLAND JULY 2013
4) CHALLENGE ROTH JULY 2015

I have split my story into these four events, to make it easier to follow my journey. At the end of each chapter, I enclose a GOLD, SILVER & BRONZE tip: Enjoy.

AARHUS
HALF- DISTANCE
TRIATHLON   2011

1: An Ironwoman is born

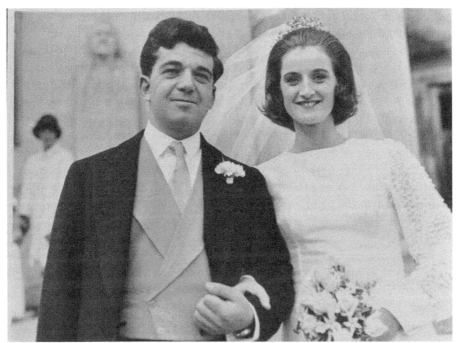

My parents on their wedding day 1964

"Dear Tiffany,

It was wonderful and sad to see you at your mother's funeral. As we did not have time to talk, I wrote down the story of how your parents, Francis and Beryl met, which as you know is also the story of how Lorraine and I met. It was in September 1963 that Francis and I went on holiday in my Ford Consul convertible, flying on a Friday night to Geneva and staying the first night in Evian on the south side of the lake. The next morning, the 21st, we set out to drive on over the pass into Italy. We had bought wine, fruit, ham, cheese and bread in the local market for a picnic lunch. We were on our way for the Great St Bernard Pass, when we passed two young ladies hitching a lift. Francis was driving and did not stop, but I said, "you should have picked them up, it's only a few miles to the big road junction and half the traffic will not be going their way". Francis swung round in a U-turn, tracked back and drew up alongside them, whereupon one of them

said, "I bet you're not going where we're going". We weren't, they wanted Chamonix. We explained that they were not hitching in a sensible place because the roads divided up ahead, so we'd give them a lift up to the junction. That car had a bench front seat, which was just as well since the back seats and the boot were full of luggage (mainly belonging to Francis). Anyway we all managed to squeeze in on the front seat and off we set. When we got to the junction we suggested that the girls might like to come up into the mountains a little way for a picnic lunch and then we would bring them back down and put them on the right road. The first nice picnic site was over the border in Italy, lunch took some time. As we packed up one of the girls said "we're not going to Chamonix, then!" and they didn't. The idea had been to find work in Chamonix and they thought that Rome might be a good alternative, so we made our leisurely way to Rome and left them there whilst Francis and I went on, as planned, to Positano. On the way back we stopped off to see how they were doing. I think Beryl had found a post for a few days as nursemaid to some ambassador's kids, Lorraine had found nothing. But they were not happy, because most work on offer as private nurses seemed to involve "droits de seigneur". So we set off again, four in the front, for St Moritz since the prospects for work there were assumed to be better. Still you know all this and I could go on for ever recalling bits and pieces, so I will just say that when Lorraine and I got engaged, my Mother reported the fact to the local paper, as one did in those days. She concluded her brief report of our engagement with the phrase "the couple met on holiday in Switzerland". Strictly true, I suppose but hardly the whole truth.
Regards, John."

Swiss-Italian border: 50 years later.

It was a gorgeous day. Lake Como was glistening in the early morning sunshine. The six of us sped past beautiful buildings, jostled with local delivery vans and bumped over the cobblestones. By the end of the day, my five biking friends and I had covered 90km on the narrow, well-worn Roman roads. As we pedalled along in single file, I could not help reflecting on my life. My parents were especially on my mind. I kept touching my mother's wedding ring, which I was wearing on a chain around my neck. They had met so close to here. My mother, originally from Northern England, had moved to Wales, then to Ghana, then to Oxford. My father came from Polish and German stock, families of scientists, musicians and law professors. He had lived in London, and then Cambridge and their paths literally crossed, almost down the road from here, in Switzerland. What if Francis had not listened to John and not turned back? That was my butterfly moment. I am the oldest of three. We grew up in England. We had a carefree existence, playing in the rolling hills of the countryside

16

from dawn to dusk, with long summers on ponies and holidays on an island in Scotland without electricity. I tried my hand at every sport offered, from fencing to Modern Pentathlon, from lacrosse to squash. I was good enough at them to play at County level, not a spectacular athlete but always gave 100%. Our bountiful youth was tragically interrupted one November day when my father died very unexpectedly at the age of 46. 17 is a young age to learn not to take anything for granted, especially people you love. Not surprisingly, I screwed up my 'A' Levels, which I had to take 6 months after his death. As I started to pick up the pieces, I found myself explaining my situation to the director of the European Business School in London and was offered a place to study Business with French and German. Four years later, I emerged with a 2:1 degree in one hand and a handsome Dutchman in the other. He went to work in the Netherlands and I in the City of London trading Eurobonds. After two years, we married and I moved to Amsterdam. I worked another 2 years trading Dutch and German government bonds. I loved this job. We traded large amounts of money; we were all young and fast. This was the late 80's early 90's. We travelled business class, had liquid lunches and it was a man's world. On the trading floor of a couple of hundred traders, there were maybe five female traders. I felt special, clever and on top of my game. In those days I was the chief earner. Roland and I did want a family and we knew we would be moving from the Netherlands some time soon with his job, therefore I knew this was not to last.

I quit in October 1991, when Sacha was born. A year later we moved to the USA. I was pregnant with a set of twins when we moved. We lost those twins when I was 6 months along. It was a heart wrenching moment when, on Christmas day 1992, we found out they had died inside me. A second hit, a loss of two more people we had loved enormously but never had the chance to get to know. Life's knocks can either take you down or sow seeds of strength.

You can either learn to dig deep and find out who you are or become overwhelmed. Triathletes are no strangers to digging deep. We lived in North America for 13 years and probably because of our twins and some other more complicated irrational reasons, ended up having four more children. We knew that if we moved to the USA, it would mean that I would not be able to be gainfully employed. This did give me the opportunity to dedicate my time and energy to raising our children, I feel very fortunate to have had this opportunity, which might not have been the case had we remained in Europe. During these child-rearing years, my interest in running was awakened. The company Roland worked for in Minnesota was a primary sponsor of the annual town marathon and half marathon. Trying to get my post-pregnancy body back into something smooth and tight, I worked out at the local

YMCA. They had three lovely women in the nursery looking after the babies and toddlers whilst the mothers attended aerobics. On Mondays, Wednesdays and Fridays, I would see a group of fit guys either intensely sprinting around the inside track or running outside in packs during their lunch hour. They were known at the "Y" as the hard-core runners, those training for the marathon. I admired them from the safety of my aerobics class. They were so cool, a little arrogant but I could not help but be in awe of their dedication, discipline and tight bellies. The moment that I decided to attempt my first half marathon did not come completely out of the blue; it had been quietly festering. I was taking some evening classes at the local university, when I met a young man who was training for his first half marathon. For some reason I figured if he could do it, I could. That did not make any sense whatsoever, given he was half my age and somewhere around his biological prime, but somehow I signed up. I dropped my YMCA membership and organised a babysitter for two hours three times a week, so I could train. I loved being outside instead of at the gym and I enjoyed the movement of running. For my first 21.1km half marathon in 1993, I decided to power walk the first half and run the second. I was so scared of the distance and not being able to finish. It took me 2 hours and 43 minutes. The following year I ran the whole thing in 2 hours and 16 minutes. It felt incredible. The fifth one, in 1997, I completed in 2 hours and 12 minutes, all the more amazing as I was still breast-feeding Natasja, daughter number three, 24/7.

 The half became my annual challenge. I was now in awe of my own dedication, discipline and not so tight but not too bad belly. I even ran a 5 km race, a month after giving birth to Tobias, number four. Life was crazy busy, but running was giving me energy and in some way helping me to straighten my body out after each pregnancy and breast-feeding stint. When Aleks arrived, five years after number four, Tobias, I had no option but to push through with bath-time, spelling homework or midnight nursing whether I was physically exhausted or not. Running helped. Our children have given us many gifts but certainly, one I appreciate daily is the gift of endurance. Those were hectic, happy years and they continued when we moved to Spain in 2005. It was in Madrid in 2009, when I finally had my body back for my own personal use that I had the guts to run my first full marathon. The feeling of accomplishment on crossing the finish line was more powerful than I had ever imagined it would be. My legs had carried me over 42,2 kilometres, now I was in awe of my own body. This was truly a dream come true. I had trained (on my own) to a level I had never expected my body or mind to attain. I felt strong, body and mind strong. I sensed that more was to come, but I had no idea how much more.
April 2010

The full distance triathlon pull started because my son Aleks (7 at the time,) was assigned to buddy Kirsten's son, Emil (recently moved from his native Denmark,) on his first day of school in Madrid. So excited with his new friend, Aleks invited him to our house and Emil whose English at the time was close to non-existent dragged his mother, Kirsten along. We drank tea and exchanged life stories. A few weeks later, Kirsten and I found ourselves sitting next to each other at a school lunch. We discussed the Madrid marathon, which I was attempting for the second time and other sporting interests we had in common. Ignoring the chatter of the 30 other women around us, we descended into our own world and tentatively I launched the crazy idea of a half distance triathlon. I had been thinking about triathlon and when a personal trainer friend of mine told me that there was a half distance triathlon or as it is sometimes known, the long course triathlon, I just could not get the idea out of my head. The sheer audacity of such a challenge dug inside my bone marrow. The distances, the unknown and the fear of taking on such an ordeal were so enormous that I was having trouble resisting the idea. Kirsten and I decided that we would mull the idea over the summer vacation and in September would determine if the idea had any merit whatsoever.

September 2010

I spent much of the summer vacation tossing over the triathlon in my mind. The numbers just seemed outrageous. The most I had ever cycled was 16km. Swimming, it had been a while, but my shoulders were still broad from a lot of swimming between the ages of eight and 15. Running, I knew I could do it but not with all that swimming and biking beforehand. The kids started back at school and I think I had resolved that it was a ridiculous challenge, way out of my comfort zone and well beyond my physical capabilities. What I did not realise then was that it was way within my mental capabilities. We met at school and Kirsten was beaming, she had that "bring on the challenge," look in her eyes. I could not fight it, I buckled, I said that I too was ready for this half distance challenge; her burning ambition was hard to resist. At our international school in Madrid, we live in something of a bubble. Most mornings, many mothers can be found in the cafeteria exchanging experiences. This informal gathering is a rich source of information for our expat. community. Every morning Kirsten dropped off her kids and went for a coffee. If you make a crazy idea such as this public, then it is harder to back out. The pressure of others knowing increases the push to train because the public shame of failure is harsh. Maybe this is why Kirsten began to talk about our plans. It became common knowledge that we were going to attempt this half distance triathlon. It did not take long before Kirsten talked to Maria and another

Dane, Anja. They were on board. Our first Tri moment took place at Kirsten's house. Armed with two computers, we started a word document titled, "half marathon.doc," it just seemed too presumptuous to call it half triathlon. I think we were in denial or something, not sure, anyway, by pushing the save button, we began our journey. I imagine we expected to fill this document with important information, although we had no idea what that might be. In reality it remained quite empty except for Kirsten's excel sheet of our original expected training schedule and hugely over-optimistic expenses calculations. For our first training session, we decided to meet at school on Friday of the next week and run the 4.5km to the local pool, where we would swim 20 x 25m, 500m (a few years later this became our warm up distance.) This was a huge deal because this was the first time we ever did two disciplines, running and swimming, together. We felt like triathletes for the first time. Next time we decided to take our goggles with us to the pool, our eyes were smarting.

November 2010

We organised our lives, children, husbands and obligations such that we could train regularly. We set up our routine, we trained (Pilates, running) on our own Mondays through Thursdays and continued to meet on Fridays, exchanging new knowledge and revelling in our new found friendship and common goal. We felt hard-core, like the YMCA guys and finally I felt my belly tightening. My friends and I were entering into a new realm, a new sisterhood.

22 November 2010

We slowly began to believe that we could do this, but we needed proper bikes. Maria already had a road bike, but all I had was my children's heavy, rusty mountain bikes and Kirsten only had her kids' little bikes. Enter Chloë, my awesome sister and her husband, Ian. As it happens Chloë and Ian are experienced road bikers. A fun time for them is ascending the Mont Blanc à la Tour de France. They came to Madrid. Kirsten, Chloë, Ian and I visited three bike stores and here began our education on bikes. Until that day, all bikes literally looked the same to us. We saw loads of bikes and became confused and realised we needed to do some research. Specifically, we had to decide which type of bike to purchase, a road bike or a TT bike. It became quite clear that this was not a cheap piece of equipment. "Overcoming obstacles" becoming our new mantra, we planned to buy our bikes after Christmas taking advantage of a New Year's discount of up to 30%. We went home and read up on bikes, fits, pedals, gears, and girlie saddles.

21 December 2010

As our training load increased in small increments we felt ready to try our first triathlon. So before the kids were finished with school for the Christmas vacation, we devised our own private triathlon with just us four as participants.

In the pouring rain we biked to the pool, swam 1.5km and started on a 20km bike circuit. Kirsten and I were on the two aforementioned heavy mountain bikes with dodgy brakes and low saddles. Anja and Maria had proper road bikes, which were not exactly perfect for the wet slippery conditions either. (It rains maybe 20 days a year in Madrid, why 21 December?) We completed the 20km, had a quick cup of tea at T2, (transition between a discipline, e.g. T1 transition between swimming and running and T2, transition between biking and running.) at my house to warm us up and then left for a 10km run. It was slowly drying and steam was rising from the roads as we crossed our own finish line. The four of us had completed our first triathlon, we were so proud of ourselves. Our smiles cracked our faces in two. We high-fived, we danced in the street; we picked up the kids with a new air of purpose. I did not record how long it took us to complete our first triathlon. We were so pumped, within three months; we had embraced the triathlon way of life. We would never look back.

We were loving this new found sport, our new friendship and the physical barriers, which we were so easily breaking down. Training together was both fun and motivating, no one wanted to be left behind. We talked about the enormity of our goals and the craziness of the full distance or ultra distance, its other name, triathlon. We finished each training session with "I would never have done it without you." We sincerely meant that.

GOLD: It is definitely easier to start on a triathlon adventure with a group of friends or a club. Go out and find similar minded friends with whom you can discover triathlon. Check out social media and find a community there.

SILVER: Be brave talk about your new found interest in triathlon. You will be amazed how many people are already doing Tri and how they want to talk about it, you will learn a lot.

BRONZE: Look up events near you, which you can go and watch or even volunteer at OR better still, sign up and do one, a small one, a short one, tell no one and just go and try it out OR organise your own private tri.

2: Obsessive

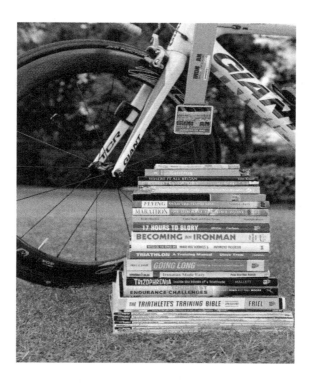

I became a little obsessed. I read everything I could lay my hands on. I pored over photos of ultra distance triathletes in magazines and training books. Particularly thrilling were photos of athletes crossing the finishing line. One I remember well was a grainy black and white photo of a finisher at the end of the book I have since lost. The look on that athlete's face was mesmerising. This was a photo of Jane Tomlinson finishing the 2003 Gatorade Half Ironman UK Champion. The image of this face I took with me on many training runs and long bike rides. Whoever this woman was, her determination was contagious. I could not lay my finger on it but she exuded in that photo what I was striving for. It was not until a lot later when I read the story of Jane Tomlinson that I realised what an incredible feat of strength finishing this race was and what an amazing athlete Jane was. She ran IRONMAN Florida whilst terminally ill with cancer. Sadly she died in 2007, but not before she raised, £1.85 million for charity.

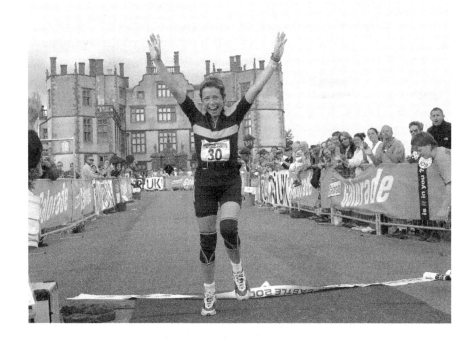

Jane Tomlinson CBE
(N.B. This is a good finishing photo.)

I read "Where it all began: The 1978 Hawaiian Ironman Triathlon," Tom Knoll tells the story of the origins of IRONMAN. He recounts the famous moments when John Collins set down the challenge of the new event to 15 competitors. It was a test of the three toughest disciplines combined. The first competition would take place on 18 February 1978 on Hawaii. He concluded his address with the words, and challenge, that anyone who could do this "would be called an Iron Man and would have bragging rights for the rest of their lives." When the race started they had no idea if anyone would be able to finish the entire Iron Man course and if they did how long it would take. It was an audacious, crazy idea and the lure was that it was tough, long and required strength, endurance and determination.

I was falling. I wanted to be an ultra distance triathlete. But I realised that anyone who completes an ultra distance triathlon is nothing short of super human and I was maybe, just maybe, half a super human but I was fairly certain that I did not have in me the kind of physical and mental strength to finish an event that would give me "bragging rights for the rest of my life." I read everything I could lay my hands on. It was fascinating. The element of athlete insecurity began to "run" through a lot of the articles I came across. What I was learning and what I was beginning to understand was that, in the world of endurance athletes, there is a narrow line between self-confidence and insecurity. Kara Bazzi, the clinical director of Opal, (a Seattle eating-disorders clinic) interviewed for Runners World,[2] was referring to distance runners when she said; "There's part of them that's threatened to be average. That mentality is a strong force to reckon with."

Chrissie Wellington, the greatest female triathlete of all time admits to an insecure edge to her motivation. "I had to make the most of it; I had to make the most of me. There could be no slack, anywhere, not in my time, not in my head, not across my skin. If there were any, the guilt wouldn't bear thinking about." — Chrissie Wellington, A Life Without Limits: A World Champion's Journey. Part of what drove me, and others which is clear in the survey of my tri-sisters is that not only are we competitive but completing an ultra distance triathlon helps us confront our insecure selves. By engaging on a challenge as brave as a full distance triathlon, our fears, wants and dreams can be somewhat fed if we accomplishing this goal. This achievement in turn gives us (enormous) confidence and satisfaction. I was aware that I craved this confidence because in my case, the insecurity of not achieving enough continually tugs away at that confidence. Testing my limits, running marathons was increasing my confidence. Setting these goals and achieving them was a heady mixture of confidence building and personal satisfaction. Also the battle between eating and exercise is constantly being waged in my head. This battle was an old friend I had known from about the age of 14. The sense was that doing triathlon would once and for all solve these two issues and simultaneously deliver a 6-pack. I could hardly wait to get going. I came across a fascinating article by professional triathlete, Ben Greenfield. In his article[3], he discusses why we "really" do triathlons. He states that we have both rational motivators for doing triathlons and irrational motivators. But what is super interesting about this is that it is the irrational motivators, which keep us training. It is not the "logical motivators for doing triathlon: improve your health, less stress, good role model, balanced lifestyle, more energy" which get us out the door week after week, come sun or rain. Rather, it is our irrational fears, desires and wants. According to Greenfield, these include: "Being able to wear your ultra distance triathlon race t-shirt in public to impress people. Being able to eat whatever you want, but not having the control, so finding a sport where working out too much is OK. Being able to fit into whatever style of clothes you wish. Having nice legs and feeling confident when you put on spandex. Telling people at parties that you're an athlete, maybe even that you have completed IRONMAN Switzerland or Florida or whichever one. Enjoying comments like, "You're really slim. Do you workout?" When trying on clothes in a store and the assistant says, "you look well trained." Some are Greenfield's examples but some are mine. All this implies discipline to me and these slide right into my motivators. I found myself fervently nodding as I read. I do enjoy responding that I do long distance triathlon and then waiting for the look of disbelief, admiration and jealousy escape from a new face before they can control it. And the favourite moment, "so how long is the full distance triathlon?" " 180 km on the bike and then a full marathon at the end?" It was all making so much sense to me; I was this type of person. It was a little uncomfortable admitting it to myself but it was definitely those irrational motivators, which drove me. I did feel a little awkward wearing my Madrid marathon t-shirts out in public since it became abundantly apparent to me that I was looking for recognition if I wore them, so for a short while I used them as pyjamas.

In Part 2, chapter 19, Can I be an ironwoman? I have included the responses of my fellow IRONMAN Zürich finishers to the question, "What motivated you to take on the IRONMAN challenge?" I also left a space for you to note down what might motivate you to take on an Ironman or half distance triathlon challenge?"

On a more mainstream level though, once again Chrissie Wellington's wise observations made me feel less wary of my irrational self. We "compete" to be the best we can in whatever we do. To quote Chrissie Wellington, again from her book, "A Life without Limits, A World Champion's Journey," "whatever you do, do it well even if it just loading the dishwasher." This is a mantra I strive to live by. I gain enormous satisfaction from completing a task well. This can be sweeping out the garage or making the speech at my brother's wedding. I would bet that this "do-it-well, do it to the extreme" element is deeply embedded in any triathlete's persona and has a profound impact on our daily lives. In all seriousness and honesty, it is probably part of the reason why we have five children. "5, amazing, how do you manage 5?" Love that! For sure for me it was the sheer audacity of undertaking such a goal. I wanted people to say "wow" when I told them what I was doing with my time. Maybe it was driven by a feeling of insecurity, at not having a job title any more other than "mom," but it was a strong force, which burned inside me and it drove me to train hard. One of the Zürich triathletes wrote, "I read that full distance triathletes are highly insecure, always seeking approval. I asked fellow full triathletes, they all agreed; we are just continually striving to be better individuals." This resonated strongly with me; I recognized this in myself. Also these words from another Zürich sister, "I needed a big challenge. I'd done marathons before and a friend of mine advised me to step into triathlon. Almost everybody thought I was nuts when I said I wanted to do the full distance...that challenged me even more." For me the dream had to be big enough to fill the hole created by the mixture of lack of self-confidence and the powerful desire to achieve something big. As I am now about to take on my first Ultra-marathon I am not sure that I will ever actually emerge from that hole.

Andrew Cherwenka estimates[4] that 700,000 people have completed an ultra distance triathlon. With a population of 7 billion, then 0,01% have completed a WTC IRONMAN. I guestimate that if you include the Challenges and Extreme Man (ultra distance triathlons run by organisations other than the World Triathlon Corporation/IRONMAN) plus other independent ultra distance triathlons it might be about 900,000 athletes who have completed an ultra distance triathlon. Calculating that female participation on average globally is about 18%,[5] then it would be about correct to guestimate that approximately 162,000 women have completed an ultra distance triathlon, thus perhaps 0.002% of earth's inhabitants are female ultra distance triathlon finishers. According to an article in ELLE magazine [6], over the past four years, "international women's registrations in full distance races have grown a whopping 275 per cent." Female participation in ultra distance triathlons is on the rise and we are loving it.

GOLD:
Consider your rational and irrational motivators. Use the table in Chapter 19 and write them down and develop them over time.

SILVER: On a run, use the alone time to analyse yourself, your strengths and weaknesses.

BRONZE: Consider how you go about your daily tasks. What might be your mantra for life?

3: Start Sweating

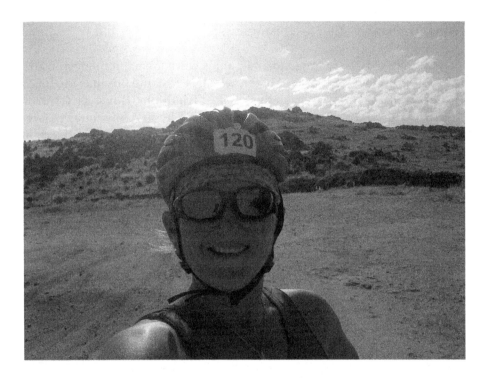

120 km solo bike ride in 32°C

11th January 2011

Not really knowing 100% what we were doing, Kirsten and I went to one of the three bike stores in our area. We chose this one because they offered the greatest discounts. We sat on a bunch of bikes, wobbled and made lame jokes. All I remember was that the seat felt very uncomfortable. The guys at the store were helpful, but I think they thought we had a screw lose. We bought two GIANT bikes and left, happy but with no real clue what lay ahead of us. The bikes turned out to be perfect, but that was more luck than judgment. This we potentially should have done differently, e.g. I should definitely have tried out a few bikes first...or maybe not!! Looking back, we probably should have bought Tri-bikes instead of road bikes, because we never did any pure bike races. Tri Bikes are only for use in triathlon competitions. Road bikes are permitted in Duathlons or other just biking events. Tri Bikes are not.

I grew up in the countryside in England and ponies were my main mode of transport to get to friends' houses. I was not a good biker, which is a shame because the bike part is obviously the largest and longest discipline of most triathlons. However I was determined to learn. I am still a very mediocre biker. The first few times we went biking I wore a trainer-shoe on my left foot and the proper bike shoe on the right foot. Being clamped into my pedals scared me.

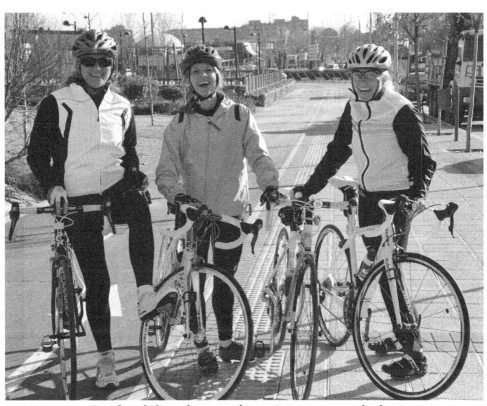
Our first bike ride, spot the trainer on my right foot

Our first bike ride was 44km. It became quite apparent that Kirsten was chief biker. From age 8 she was biking 6 km to school and back every day and from 17, she biked 10 to 20 km to get to school and activities. She had not told us that before we went out. Not that we were competitive or anything. I think at this point it would be fair to say that we were no longer working out; we were training. This was a major transition. We began to think about nutrition and hydration in a whole new way. We did feel we could eat more, which is always a bonus and if we were honest, partly why we were in this game in the first place. We learned that if we attempted a longer distance without having prepared properly then it was much harder. This meant drinking lots of water the night before and starting the ride well hydrated. It soon became evident that we were unable to undertake longer bike rides, say 60km without eating well before hand. I remember when we covered 58 km for the first time I felt I had a small chance at 90 km. Maria, Anja and Kirsten were always patient, waiting for me at the last junction where we turned off the bike path and onto the main road. Anja would always shout with a grin, "ready for the last 5." Of course we were always ready for the last 5 km. These were our first outings, which were longer. This was the beginning of our mental training. We were feeling tired legs and learning to push through that discomfort. Being ready for the last five meant that we had won the mental battle for that particular work-out because we were on the home stretch. I remember the feeling I had in the last 11 km of IRONMAN Switzerland marathon, it was the knowledge that I had won the mental battle, after fighting it for 14 hours and that I could relax and finish IRONMAN Switzerland. The mental battle is the understanding simultaneously that you are in pain or tired but that you still have the grit to finish. It is the devil and angel on your shoulder syndrome. Understanding your pain helps you to push on through. Knowing that the pain is derived from tired, grumpy muscles allows you to wrestle with your head and win. On the other hand if the pain is more serious, an injury developing, then it is time to stop.

March 25th /26th 2011

We decided it was time to try an open water swim. This was a harrowing experience. We three girls, Maria, Kirsten and I took the train to sweltering 36ºC Valencia. Maria's biggest fear was us three getting lost in the ocean and never being found again. She brought a pink blow up dolphin belonging to her daughter, Klara and two balloons and some ribbon.

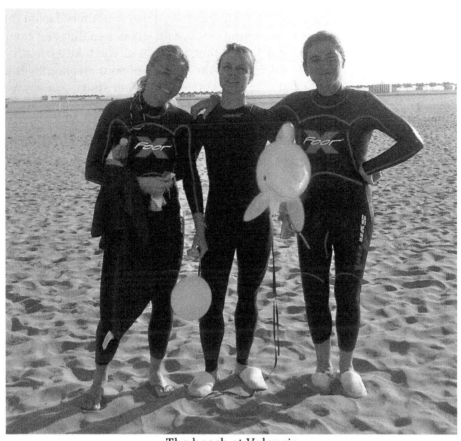
The beach at Valencia

I went to the beach feeling that swimming was my strongest discipline, the only one in which I had any advantage over the other two. We donned our wetsuits, hats, goggles, dolphins and balloons and launched ourselves amid giggles and nervousness. The waves were unforgiving. We started off swimming with the current. We swam maybe 100 meters and I was hit by fear. It is hard to describe this fear, but I think it is connected to claustrophobia. Later I learned more about it in an effort to overcome it, but at this particular moment it was a completely unexpected response to being in the water.   Maria, the weakest swimmer, was enjoying the extra buoyancy that the salt water gave her. She had worried, that once in the water, she would be cold, specifically her face, but this was not happening and she felt very reassured. We continued on, with the current and I felt I could control the fear rising in my chest. But when we decided to test our skills against the current we were confronted by waves at unexpected angles and frequencies, which obviously had never bothered us in the pool. Good swimming technique is breathing on the odd strokes so that you can be aware of what is happening on your right and then left side as you take a breath. In bumpy water this is much harder and you lose the rhythm of your stroke. Swimming in open water, we were learning fast was a completely different sport. I guess we had been really naïve about this, and it shows how little we had really read around the subject of triathlon because there is a lot of tri-literature dedicated to the swim. We ploughed on for another 200 meters; I was suffering. I pride myself on breathing every 3 strokes. This type of breathing was serving no purpose as the waves were slamming into me on one side. Also the constant push of the tide made me feel sick, totally disorientated and like a boat without a rudder. I hung in the water, seasick, scared, with a very salty mouth feeling like I was going to throw-up.

Kirsten took on the leadership role and dragged me out of the water so I could catch my breath. Fully clad in our hot, unflattering wetsuits, we emerged from the waves onto the beach. The gorgeous, fashionable Spanish sun worshippers could not help but gaze in surprise as we dragged ourselves up the beach. It did look as if we had swum quite a distance to arrive on those shores. At this time we did not have our cool triathlon waterproof watches so we did not really have any idea of how far we had swum so we based our calculations on the time we had been in the water, about 35 minutes. It was not that far and it was super demoralising for me at least. We decided that we would have to swim again the next morning before catching our train home. That evening before dinner we walked the beach. Using a running watch we estimated the distance on land and set ourselves landmarks so that we would be able to gauge the distance when swimming the next day. The following morning the waves were much calmer which did ease my fear but I knew I had a lot of work ahead of me. What was interesting about this humbling experience was how much we were learning about ourselves; who we were and how we were responding to the training. These lessons were not always comfortable. Training for an ultra triathlon is so much more than training for an ultra triathlon; it is very much a mind game. Positive mind; and you feel strong, negative mind; you doubt your ability. The psychology is intense; the emotions go up and down, so learning how to deal with yourself, physically and mentally is a fun ride, especially if you record your emotions and read over them some time later.

GOLD: Keep a record of how much water you are drinking in a day, and how well you are feeling when you are training. Monitor energy levels and general level of enjoyment.

SILVER: Pain can be your friend. Get to know and understand your different types of pain. Some pain you should push through, other pain, definitely not. This is the beginning of mental training.

BRONZE: If you feel seasick in the water, do 6 somersaults in a row every day and eat ginger.

4: Pen and Paper or Excel sheet: you need a plan

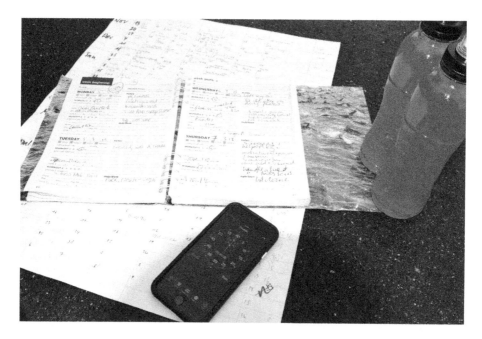

My training diary

Training for the full distance triathlon will only work if you have a plan. And on those occasions when you cannot follow the plan you have to be flexible. This flexibility in itself is part of the plan as it is good training for a triathlon race because if something unexpected happens on race day you need to be able to deal with it without crumbling into a weeping heap. For our first half distance in Aarhus, Denmark, the water was so cold, 13.8º C that we were only permitted to swim one km; nobody missed having the opportunity to swim the second kilometre. Conversely, in Zürich in 2013, the water was so warm we were not permitted a wetsuit. We had never swum so far in open water without a wetsuit. What you might expect to go wrong will not. On running his first half distance in Spain, a friend worried for weeks about the heat, having done most of his training in rainy Belgium. Turned out that his biggest problem on the day of the race was stomach issues. He drank tap water in Madrid for the last few days before the race and it upset his stomach. In his words, "be prepared for the slim chance you might have to change your goal half-way through the race; mine went from finishing in a decent time, to just making it to the finish line." The plan has four functions:

1) It augments your fitness over a certain period of time to bring you to peak fitness for race day, hopefully whilst avoiding injury.
2) It helps you make the most use of your training time and
3) It allows you to schedule time for your work and family.
4) A plan will settle your nerves. It will not stop you waking up in the middle of the night with the deeply nagging thought that we all ask ourselves constantly, "Am I training enough? Am I training too much? Am I training right?" It will enable you to remind yourself that you are following a plan probably in part written by someone who has either completed an ultra triathlon or is a professional coach. If you write down the distances you train it will settle your nerves (a little.) Crossing the line of a full distance triathlon is a testimony to an athlete's time management and effective training. The women who complete an ultra distance triathlon are physically and mentally strong and also masters of time management. All the books and trainers tell you to set your ABC races. Your A races are your big goals; usually you will have one in a season or year. The B races are training races; you might have three, hopefully at least one swim, one run and one bike. The C races are practices, rich learning grounds, maybe shorter distances, you expect to finish but not in a fast time. They are for nutrition, gear, race nerves and pace experimentation. You might have three to five of these. Working backwards from your A race, you plan your training, your vacations, your life and your B and C races. There are plenty of plans available on the Internet and in books. Chose one that works for you and tailor it to your life. For my second full distance triathlon, I basically trained on my own. I set my own targets based on the training plans in Christina Gandolfo's great book, "The Woman Triathlete." There is also much information about ABC races available. This is the most fun part of training for an ultra distance triathlon as you set out all your goals for the training period starting from the ultra triathlon and working backwards. Below you can see all the races I have done on the road to the two full distance triathlons I have completed. You see how the Buitrago half distance 2012 was an A race and became a B when completed in 2015. Then it is fun to look back and see if you complete these races faster or slower as you age!!

See below in chronological order:

DATE	LOCATION	RACE	A, B OR C	MY TIME
1993-2005	Duluth, MN, USA	8 x ½ marathons		2:43 to Personal best: 1:52
April 2009	Madrid, Spain	Marathon	A	4:16
April 2010	Madrid, Spain	Marathon	A	4:12
2 April 2011	Madrid, Spain	1/2 marathon	C	1:55
17 April 2011	Madrid, Spain	Marathon	B	3:58 personal best
5 June 2011	Salou (Barcelona)	Extreme Man	Maria A	
3 July 2011	**Aarhus, Denmark**	**½ distance tri**	**A**	**6:25**

DATE	LOCATION	RACE	A, B OR C	MY TIME
6 August 2011	Wisconsin, USA	3.2km Point–la Pointe swim	C	1:23
1 April 2012	Madrid, Spain	½ marathon	C	
15 April 2015	Vienna, Austria	Marathon	B	4:01
12 May 2012	**Buitrago, Spain**	**½ distance tri**	**A**	**6:55**
7 July 2012	Buelna, Spain	½ distance tri	(Kirsten & Maria) A	6:06

DATE	LOCATION	RACE	A, B OR C	MY TIME
4 August 2012	Wisconsin, USA	3.2 km Point-la Pointe swim	C	1:21
7 April 2013	Madrid, Spain	½ marathon	C	1:57
28 April 2013	Madrid, Spain	Marathon	B	4:18
2 June 2013	Zürich, Switzerland	90 km bike loop	B	
28 July 2013	**Zürich, Switzerland**	**IRONMAN SWITZERLAND**	**A**	**15:02**

DATE	LOCATION	RACE	A, B OR C	MY TIME
3 November 2013	New York, USA	Marathon	C	4:25
6 April 2014	Madrid, Spain	½ marathon	C	
27 April 2014	Madrid, Spain	Marathon	B	4:37
3 August 2014	Wisconsin, USA	3.2km Point–la Pointe Swim	C	1:16
8 February 2015	Madrid, Spain	El Pardo ½ marathon	C	2:08
8 March 2015	Cambridge, England	½ marathon	C	2:35
13 June 2015	Buitrago, Spain	½ distance tri	B	6:42
5 July 2015	Roth, Germany	90km bike loop	B	
12 July 2015	**Roth, Germany**	**DATEV** CHALLENGE **ROTH**	**A**	**14:58**

DATE	LOCATION	RACE	A, B OR C	MY TIME
10 April 2016	Rome, Italy	Marathon	B	4:40
10 September 2016	Jungfrau, Switzerland	Marathon	A	5:55
30 October 2016	Luzern, Switzerland	Marathon	A	4:16
1 July 2017	Zermatt Switzerland	Mountain ½ Marathon	A	3:11

The distances you train and times really depend on your own life, but however you work it, a training log, calendar and planning are essential. In the questionnaire I asked how the Zürich women managed to juggle commitments and fit their training into the lives. Their responses are in Chapter 23; Sharpen your pencils, let's make a plan. As time goes by, you get to know your body better. This is an exciting journey. You learn what you need to do to prepare for a tougher training day. A day or two before a long bike ride I know that my head will start whining about the 6 hours of hard work that lie before me. I know that my left hamstring is the first muscle to start tightening up as my training becomes more intense. I also know that if I can get out the door especially in cold temperatures and push my body to run the first two kilometres I usually feel an intense thrill of being alive and profound happiness as I trot through my local woods for a fun 10 km run. Natascha Badmann, in her book "9 Stunden zum Ruhm," "9 Hours to Fame," explains that she takes her basal temperature every morning and based on that reading, trains hard or less hard that day. Many world-class athletes in any discipline record their waking body temperature. A change by more than 0.5 to 1°F or 0.28-0.55°C is a possible indication of overtraining, and thus the intensity or duration of a scheduled workout might be reduced until the waking temperature is back to the baseline. That is what is required to be world-class athlete. An amateur needs to listen to her body and how it is responding to training but should not need to take basal temperature. Listening to the body is a crucial element of training because it is an important step in avoiding injury. Nothing will upset you more than injuring yourself such that you have to stop training. Then your head goes into overdrive and your mental balance deteriorates rapidly. The key is juggling commitments and listening to your body, being flexible with your plan and noticing improvement. Different people organise their lives in different ways. Some join Tri Clubs, which is a tremendous boost to organising your training; others rely on FB or join other social media groups or Strava etc., experiment and see what works for you.

GOLD: Record all your training and at the end of the week add up the distances and hours spent on all disciplines. Specifically, compare intended training session and actual training session. This way you will learn to be flexible in a week's training.

SILVER: Become informed on your anatomy; learn about muscles and fascia, the skeleton and cartilage. Record any aches and pains so you can see if a pattern is developing.

BRONZE: Train with a friend or SMS your training plans frequently to a friend if you can, so that s/he can see when you are over-training or pushing an injury too far and s/he can tell you to stop. Sometimes you need someone else to give you permission to slow down.

5: Bring it on; we are ready

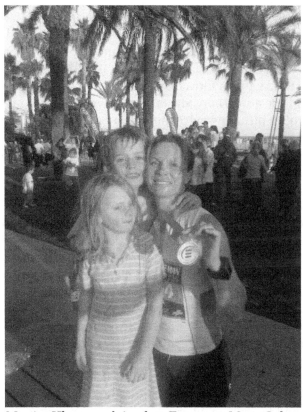

Maria, Klara and Axel at Extreme Man, Salou
(Sorry about quality, only photo we have of this moment)

January 2011

In early January, the day before we bought our bikes, we had decided to sign up for a
half distance triathlon: Challenge Aarhus in Denmark on 3 July 2011. We chose Aarhus
for four reasons. 1) the dates worked 2) because Kirsten has family in Denmark 3) my
husband had a cousin there with whom we could stay and 4) all my Danish friends

promised me Denmark was a flat as a pancake. With the A race fixed we worked backwards. In preparation for this we would have a B race, the marathon of Madrid, 17 April 2011 and a C race the half marathon in Madrid on 3 April. We had no swimming or biking B or C races.

It turned out that 3 July was not a good date for Maria and her family as they had a reunion planned in Sweden for that date, so not to be outdone, and not to train for nothing, Maria sought out another A race. She signed up for the Extreme Man in Salou, in northern Spain. An Extreme Man is the full distance tri. When she told us we were shocked! To understand why an ultra distance triathlon was a doable goal for Maria you have to know a little about her. She is lean, driven, an economical runner, who spent most of her youth pursuing a dream to be a professional ballet dancer. She has abdominal muscles to die for. She gave up ballet for a degree in Economics only when she could not be the prima ballerina in her dance company. She has three children and there is not a shred of evidence on her tight little body!

Five weeks before her A race, the Salou Extreme Man, Maria decided to cycle the 180km bike portion of her Extreme Man this was to be Maria's C race. The Extreme Man organisers arranged this outing for the participants so they could see the territory. She and her husband Klaus packed their bikes and water bottles and headed up the coast towards Barcelona. With a band of 30 others, they wove their way through the Tarragona Mountains for 7 ½ hours. Afterwards, Klaus said every single part of his body ached, including his fingernails. But they had done the distance, we were astonished and proud, it was an incredible feat and a fantastic learning experience. So much for incremental training Maria had gone from 70km to 180km in a few weeks.

Whilst Maria was cycling in Salou, on the mountainous coast 110km South West of Barcelona, Kirsten and I were feeling supremely cool. We biked the 17 km into Madrid and ran a half marathon. We were chuffed at how hard-core we were becoming.

17 April 2011

Two weeks later, the three of us attempted our first B race, and Kirsten's first marathon. Kirsten and I set off together and did the first 10km in 52 minutes, we felt good, strong and excited! We had no idea where Maria was we had not seen her since

10 minutes before the start. Kirsten took off at the 10km water table and I forced myself to stick to the plan because I was running faster than ever and I knew the hardest part was always going to be the 25KM to 32km in the park. Training on Roland's stationary bike had been bugging my knee, which decided to start complaining around 22km just before the park. At 23km, I needed the bathroom so ducked into a hotel to use their bathroom. I rinsed my head under the cold-water tap as two ladies looked on and then stood aside to let me pass. One said to the other, "let her go she is in more of a hurry then we are." Stopping the momentum, my knee had totally stiffened up; so I started to walk, jog slowly to get it moving again. It bugged me for the rest of the race I just kept going one km at a time focusing on ignoring pain. I wished I had taken an ibuprofen before the race and I wished I had one in my little running belt. I was annoyed at myself because I had experimented with taking an ibuprofen during practice runs and it had alleviated the pain without causing dehydration. By 32km I had reached what was for me mentally the furthest point of the marathon, because once we rounded that point we were on the return to the city centre and heading home. Here I began to feel better until the 4-hour timing balloon passed me. Oh well I was still in the race and I was not going to accelerate now. I had a gel at 35km because I knew there was an incline ahead. I ploughed on waiting for the entrance to the Retiro Park to come into view; it took its time. I touched the wrought iron gate as I entered into the park as I had done last year and have done each year since. Finally, closing in on the finish, aerobically I felt good; it was really just my knee bugging me as I entered the last 500 metres. Before I knew it Aleks was running the last 200metres with me. Under the banner, over the mat a quick look at my watch and I realised that I had completed a personal best that stands, still to this day of 3.58. The 4-hour balloon had passed me but my net time was 3.58. I found Kirsten and Maria, both of whom looked fresh after their marathons, completed in 3.39 and 3.22 respectively. With that time Maria qualified for the New York marathon! We all felt terrific. Our training was clearly making a difference. To gain a place at the New York City Marathon, you can either run for a charity and raise a minimum amount through sponsorship, you can try through the lottery or you can run another city marathon and qualify by running under a certain time, e.g. for a 50-54 year old woman, the qualifying time is 3:51 for a marathon and 1:49 for a half in a qualifying city.

May 2011

With a marathon success in the bag we got back onto our bikes. We started racking up the distances, 63km here, 71km there sometimes we ran after, maybe a km or two. Then one day Anja and Kirsten went out and rode 100km in the baking Madrid

May heat and then ran 2.5km. Have to admit I felt a little sick on hearing that. All the time we were learning that we weren't going anywhere for any period of time unless we kept hydrated and hydrating whilst riding is a relatively easy activity on the bike. Also we were learning that eating on the bike was a skill we had to master. We have definitely dropped a few gels on the road. As we slowly took on the mantle of triathletes we were also learning about our equipment. Not that we felt remotely comfortable with it yet and there were some good lessons coming our way. However we were realising that if we were going to fail at this mission it would be our bodies, not our equipment that would let us down. We played with saddle heights, learned to pump tyres using the right valves and decided we needed better swim goggles. We invested in wetsuits, which we bought on-line and later replaced with a better one, as we trained for IRONMAN Switzerland in Zürich.

We biked as much as our children-driven schedules allowed us, always in, at least, pairs. One trip Maria and I did our usual 32km trek on the bike trail to Soto del Real and somehow got lost. We asked a pedestrian the way back to the trail. I had only my left foot out of the pedal and leaned too far to the right. I began to fall ever so slowly to the right and there was nothing I could do to stop my fall. The woman who was busy pointing directions did not notice me gracefully easing towards the pavement. She turned around and saw me at her feet. "Que pasa hija?" "What are you doing down there?" She asked. I explained my foot was caught in the pedal and she helped me up, in the mean time Maria biked back laughing so much her bike was swerving from side to side. It was a cool day and once we got back to the cars I ran 1.5 km just to test my legs, Maria went off to a lunch. Lesson learned on this ride was that you don't have to finish with a salty face. I had kept myself well hydrated by concentrating on my water intake. In fact you don't want to finish with a salty face. A salty face means you have done a bad job at keeping hydrated. If you finish the bike part of an endurance race with a hydration deficit, number one you have to be aware of that and number two you have to attend to it fast. We were beginning to learn about our own bodies and more importantly we were beginning to listen to our bodies. It was a good day I felt in control and I knew we were getting stronger.

1 June 2011

The Thursday before Salou Extreme Man 2011, we went to Maria's house for a coffee. The plan was to help her with the packing and simultaneously put together a list of all things needed for an ultra distance race. We noted everything from salty snacks to spare inner tubes; not that any of us was remotely confident in our ability to change a tire. She packed a signed good luck towel we gave her and (her maybe 6 times used) wet-suit. We visualised the event and double-checked her gear. As we were about to leave Kirsten suddenly pointed out that she had forgotten to pack her running shoes! That is how nervous she was. Maria remained fairly confident that once she had made it through the swim component she could fight her way through the rest. The swim cut off was 2 hours and that was her greatest challenge. For my part I could not fathom how anyone on our training was going to bike 180 km and then run a marathon, but that is the beauty of Maria.

5 June 2011

Maria swam a brilliant time of 1.28.55 and with that in the bag she embarked on the bike. The course she knew from her expedition with Klaus five weeks earlier. It was still hilly. Afterwards she told us it was a battle of the mind, a sheer case of pure survival. We loved to hear her story; it spoke directly to our half-distance-tri souls. I remember at home tidying up after lunch on that Sunday and Maria was on the bike portion, I remember preparing dinner and Maria was still on the bike stretch. At the time I thought, I was not made of the same proteins and calcium as my friend Maria, there was no way that my body was ever going to undertake that kind of test. The bike leg took her 8.14.23. With 9 minutes and 54 seconds in T2, she started her marathon. She completed her 42.2km run in 4 hours and 1 minute, three minutes slower than my (personal best) Madrid marathon time, how could that be? Her run was even more impressive because she had run it without the aid of music pumping in her ears. We always wore music when running, we could not imagine running any distance without the distraction of music. No i-Pods allowed for the ultra distance tri marathons. It was clear we had a lot to learn about concentration and mind-set. In time, we did master this art and now I prefer to run without music. Within five minutes of her finish, Klaus sent round a photo of a triumphant Maria. She was incredible, he wrote, "tired but beautiful." My eyes stung and tears ran down my cheeks as I looked at that photo, thinking about her courage and that she had achieved that on our little training plan. I wanted that kind of admiration from my husband! Who doesn't? She was radiant holding onto her kids with the Spanish sun setting in the background and a bright shiny full distance medal around her neck; total time 14.05, 3rd in her category. We were in awe.

Swim	1:28
Bike	8:14
Run	4:01
TOTAL	14:05

The story in Maria's words;

"*I guess the summary could be: Either you should be super prepared and that makes you calm the day before the race OR the less you know sometimes mentally is better. I had no clue what I was going into and no one expected me to make it. The morning of race day I walked to the start realising that the watch I was going to have in the water had run out of battery and I would not be able to know how long I had been swimming. Not being very good at crawling straight I decided that swimming breaststroke was most efficient. Just taking it easy and trying to get around the course, ignoring that I was last by far. Once I had done 1.5 loops, I had to ask one of the canoes following me what time it was. And I realized that I was much faster than I had expected. Getting out of the water I was sooo happy that I had managed to swim the distance so I just changed slowly and put new sun-tan lotion on and was confident that if I just now didn't overdo it I could make it. I had absolutely no problem at all finding my bike among the 5 or 6 bikes left. I had done the full loop once with my husband before which was nice because I knew the course. The time we trained they had only one arranged water/food stop by the organiser and that was way too little water and food for me. Luckily we found a gas station around 75km so we could fuel up on Red Bull and snickers before doing the last 75k as we were totally exhausted. So during the race I made sure that I filled up both drinking bottles at all stops during the race and had 2 Peanut Butter sandwiches to eat, and chocolate and bars.... i.e. I was not dehydrated and made several pee stops. But I did threw up in the evening, I don't know why but I think that was because of lack of salt, as I didn't have that problem in Zürich and there I had several salt sticks on the run. On the run I had a mouth full of water, at least, on every possibility.*"

Maria was our hero. She sowed a seed, the ultra distance seed. It just grew and grew inside us. I started wondering if I had what it took to do an ultra distance triathlon. A half (for me) was one thing, but double the distance quite something else. Who was I? What makes an endurance athlete?

GOLD: Always carry an Ibuprofen with you, whether it is a half marathon or a full distance triathlon, you never know. Experiment with the effect it might have on your performance; some say they cause dehydration. I have never noticed that.

SILVER: Most of us mortals need to build up the distances slowly, deliberately, following a plan to avoid injury. Remember, most of us cannot pull off a Maria.

BRONZE: Try and run every time after a long bike session even if it is only 2km. You will see, that with practice, your body can adapt to this demand quite easily

6: Raw sewage, cross wind, a museum: The Aarhus Half

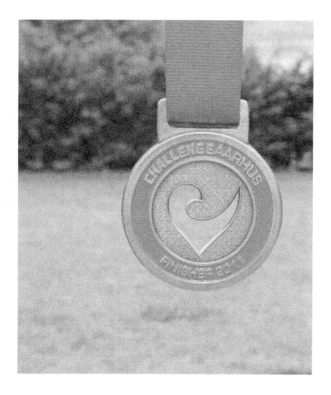

First Triathlon medal

With exactly four weeks to go we hunkered down and got focused. For the next three weeks, we decided to do one long run, one long bike and one long swim each week with two or maybe more circuit training sessions at a sport's complex as well. The circuit training sessions entailed 20 minutes on the treadmill composed of a two minute sprint followed by a two minute jog, five times, the same in the pool, 20 minutes in total with two minutes sprint, two minute relax five times and same on a stationary bike. This we repeated, thus we trained for two hours. This also honed our transition skills making us take on and off shoes, get used to biking with wet shorts and taught our legs to change disciplines quickly. We felt we were pretty much triathletes now. We slept, ate, and dreamt Aarhus. It invaded our every moment. We tried not to burden our families but when together on the bike or running we talked about it all incessantly. We concluded that the swimming was very therapeutic and kept our muscles somewhat limber. As the Madrid temperatures crept up, training became more intense but we figured this was good for us, as Aarhus would never come close to the 35ºC we were experiencing.

31 June 2011

We arrived in Aarhus a few days early and to my surprise realised that where we were staying was about a 50-minute drive from Aarhus city centre. The second unplanned event was that my bike did not arrive; it had been left in Madrid. It is hard to describe the emotions of the days in the run up to our first half distance. It is hard even to process the emotions. I ate pasta, tried to sleep well, drink well. I went on a quick bike ride to the beach on a bike way too small for me and worried that by using different muscles I would ruin all my training. I put on my wetsuit and left my clothes and bike on the deserted beach and hoped that no one would steal either of them. I took a dip in the chilly, dark, salty sea and swore under the water. It was all so outrageously scary.

Two days later my bike arrived and I set about putting it together. I felt pretty professional doing this although inside I felt far from in charge especially of the bike. We had practiced changing tyres a few times but I was still unsure how well I would do if push came to shove and if I would just burst into tears if I actually did have to deal with a puncture.

1 July, Roland and Natasja arrived, followed by Kirsten, Lars, and their two sons Emil and Jeppe. We were all staying together at Roland's cousin, Renée's house. 2 July, we boarded our rental van with mine and Kirsten's bikes, tons of gear and our 3 kids. We set off for Aarhus to register and attend the pre-race meet. We joined the other tri-athletes; that was a big moment; we joined the other tri-athletes. Our bikes passed the security check and we left them in the bike park. We strolled around the exhibitors'

tents and ate some more pasta. We had planned to stay the night in a hotel 500 metres from the start. Lars and Roland dropped us and the rest of our gear off at the hotel and left us. That was another poignant moment. Kirsten and I loaded our water bottles and grabbed her car. We wanted to drive the bike course. I tried to follow the instructions and map all written in Danish, horrifically strangling the Nordic language, as we set off into the land of the Vikings. We basically found the route, missed a few turns here and there but had something of an idea of what lay before us the day after. One of the reasons we had chosen Aarhus as half-virgins is because Kirsten and others had assured me that Denmark was flat. We soon came to realise that flat in a car is not flat on a bike and wherever she had grown up, maybe that was flat, but what lay ahead of us was definitely not flat. We stepped out of the car at one point and I noticed that there was more than a gentle breeze drifting over the cattle fields. It was time to go back to the hotel and start putting our heads in order, thinking positive thoughts and focusing on finishing.

For the two weeks up to the Challenge Aarhus half distance event the weather had been desperate in Aarhus. It had been raining a lot and we were told during the race meet on the Saturday afternoon, that maybe the swimming part of the race would have to be substituted for a 4km run. The bay where the swim would take place was also part of the town's water management system. Water management system was a nice way of saying waste management and as the drains had been overflowing too much "garbage" had leaked into the bay. If the rain subsided then the swim would take place, we would be told in the morning. Even though the race organisers were talking about sewage in the bay, I still preferred to swim than run. I guess I did not believe that the Danes would really have such a medieval system. We knew that triathlon is all about being flexible now we were experiencing it. The water temperature on July 2nd was also low. Under 14ºC, the Triathlon rules state that no swim portion of a race can be longer than one km.

3 July 2011

This was the culmination of 9 months' work. We finally went to sleep around 11pm, having checked over our equipment I don't know how many times. It turned out I had left my swim goggles on my bed at Renée's place so I had to borrow Kirsten's second pair; thank goodness she had a second pair. These were her brand new sun-filtered snazzy, reflective swim goggles perfect for the bright Spanish sun, very mediocre for early, dark Scandinavian mornings in northern Denmark. But hey they were goggles and I was grateful and whom else did I know who has two pairs of goggles. Our hotel was right on the beach so I kept waking up, sitting up in my bed, straining my neck to check if the wind was rising and if the sea was becoming choppy. We slept sporadically, arose with the first light, tried hard to eat breakfast with all the other triathletes and got ready. Sitting in that quiet breakfast room, trying hard to cram the carbs, I reflected on how frustrating it was to have the opportunity to eat as much as I could handle but feeling so sick to my stomach that I could not. I was annoyed at myself for not being able to take advantage of what was in effect a free lunch. Slowly, we triathletes paraded our way along the waterfront to the race tent to find out if we were swimming and how far. It was announced that we would swim, a relief I thought at the time and good news, only one km.

179 pink caps made up the female wave, the first Age-Groupers to start after the professionals. We descended into the water and I gasped, I realized I needed a plan, I started to panic, I did not have a swim race day plan. We stood at the back of the field. As we waited, we hugged, high-fived and tears clouded my vision, the emotion was making me tremble all over, my goggles rattled in my hand and my feet quivered in the soggy sand. It felt momentous to be at this point, as if my whole life somehow had been leading up to this moment. Everything had been preparing me for this. We were beginning this day with no idea how it would turn out. That takes guts and I guess I had not really understood until this very moment how many guts it took.

The trouble with swimming is that it is not like running you can't slow down, stop, tie your shoes laces, draw uneven breaths, touch the ground every few minutes and regroup. You can't even see where you are going most of the time. Even on the bike you can slow down, stretch, see ahead, look behind. With swimming all this is impossible. We descended into the water and I gasped, I realised again that I really needed a plan, I started to panic, I still did not have a swim race day plan. I looked around urgently. We started; I was losing it. There were people all around me plunging in. I dropped to my knees and forced my shoulders under the water, I floundered uselessly. The coarse taste of the salt on my tongue made me wretch. I looked for the outside of the pack. I stretched my arms in front of me, put my head underwater and lifted my legs. I began my front crawl stroke. I tried to find my familiar rhythm. My heart was racing; my breathing was highly irregular. My head would not let itself be dipped into the water. My head did not trust this situation and wanted to keep above the water and look around it. I could feel my pulse in my gums and temples and my rib cage felt as if it were going to break under the pressure from inside my body. I had to take control of myself, had to take back my body. I kept searching for my smooth 3x3 stroke and breathing routine but I just could not control myself, there was no way I could settle down.

Then my swim cap fell off. I stopped I wanted that cap for future swimming training prestige, (those bragging rights) I turned went against the flow, grabbed it and stuffed it down my wetsuit. Now my head was cold, my goggles were like wearing sunglasses; I forced myself onwards. It was horrible; there were jellyfish around me I kept veering off to the coastline. I was breathing 2x2 onto my right side, so had no point of reference on my left, which was where the rest of the pack was. I practically bumped into an orange rescue boat. I swam back to the heaving group of swimmers hating every single second of what I was doing. I swam breaststroke, some doggie paddle and some crawl. I was hit in the face, the sides and also collided with other people. How I made it to the half way marker, I have no idea. I was constantly talking to myself and the jellyfish around me; I was attempting to threaten both them and me. I was so angry with myself for having lost total control of a situation. When had I last been so useless?

At the marker I took the inside lane. My heart was still racing I felt like the wetsuit was suffocating me, constricting movement and breath, the exact anti-yoga state of mind. Pink caps kept passing me. I doggy-paddled/breast-stroked/ kicked my way to the second buoy and tried to keep my act together. I could see the finish now ahead of me so I told myself to swim crawl, that surely this nightmare would be over in less than 15 minutes. I told myself I could do this, anyway the only way out of this mess was to swim I reasoned. I continued to swim, veered off to the right again, my goggles steamed up I stopped to spit in them, no one was in the way because I was now officially at the very tail end of the pack and way out on the right heading out to sea. I hated being so incompetent. So scared and so much the powerless victim. Simultaneously I was aware how much mental energy I was burning. More jelly fish and then I started imagining one clamping itself to my face so I could not breathe, I fought off the image quickly. I ploughed on still doing a slow 2x2 stroke, then I caught sight of Kirsten and she shouted something about drafting to keep me from veering off. I tried but was really way too scared I just wanted to get out of the water. I looked up saw the finish line again it looked closer; I regrouped and swam some more. I saw Anja in front of me, which was super dispiriting because I was a far stronger swimmer than she. I felt sick, dizzy, but was closing in on the finish. I centred, forced my arms to crawl the last metres, pressing through seaweed and jelly fish, I laughed at them, I am getting out of here and leaving you behind you filthy animals. I exited and immediately slipped on a rock, thankfully a volunteer picked me up and I left the Danish water behind forever. A few guys from the next wave ran past me. It was 7.30am and already I had expended so much energy. I felt drained. My face was pale, my legs wobbly and my self-esteem shaken and stirred. (haha I laughed at myself.) How could my strongest discipline have gone so horribly wrong? I had been in the water all of about 25 minutes.

I ran to the bike park to look for my bike, it wasn't hard to find since there were only about 8 bikes left on the ladies' racks where earlier that morning there had been 179. I put on my helmet and started running with my bike to the start of the bike course. I had never run with my bike before, so awkwardly held onto the saddle and the handlebars simultaneously. I fumbled with my glove for what seemed like forever and decided against wearing my sunglasses, which still had their dark lenses in for Madrid riding. I had never cycled in any other conditions other than the bright Spanish sun so had not even thought about changing them. The sky was grey and my sweaty forehead was already clouding them up anyway. I was finally under way. It must have taken me about 5km to settle down on the bike. This was a pure triathlon moment; putting the swim behind me and looking forward. The ability to gather strength from her own resources is a powerful tool for any woman in any walk of life.

The course was described in the Aarhus information packet as a technical course. So-called flat Denmark, whose highest mountain is 400 metres above sea level, was lying to us. We thought our hilly training route and being 600 metres above sea level would prepare us well for whatever Aarhus and its suburbs would throw at us. Well now I know "technical" is tri-speak for hilly, narrow roads and sharp turns. I also know that strong northerly winds whip across Denmark's curvaceous countryside. Obviously you do not place plenty of windmills where there is no wind. Last night these very same windmills looked cute and rustic, now they were just getting on my nerves.

I rode the first 30km uphill constantly on the look out for the relaxing, gratifying down hills to stretch my legs. I hit the 50km on my meter and kept waiting for the biking high, the raw feeling of being alive, the one that during training had propelled me forward. It felt like I just went uphill and uphill and more uphill. It seemed to me that of the 90km maybe 7km were downhill, I still cannot figure out how that worked. To keep me going I looked at the names and nationalities of the tight little butts which kept passing me. There must have been more than 1,000 riders who overtook me. Most were Danish; there were many Mads, Christians, Peters and Clauses. 3 Brits passed me, 5 Germans, a Pablo, a Mark a Phil or two, a Brazilian, an American, many gallantly urged me forward. I was never in pain; I kept my breathing constant and just ploughed on and on and on. As we went through villages I looked for new Danish words and said "morn" to the inhabitants, all this kept me going and helped me repair my ravaged post-swim self-esteem. My dumb sunglasses fell out of my back pocket twice! My chain jumped off but my tires remained in tact. I saw many flats on the way,

53

maybe 20 or so. Three and a half hours later, I came down the hill to the harbour; I even overtook a lady and closed in on the finish. Tears sprang to my eyes, it is not easy to bike and cry and I had not had much practice.

My lips and face were salty. I was not sure if this was due to the horrible swim, sweat or tears. I tried to keep drinking during the ride but did not even finish the 2 litres of my Camelbak. I had merely drunk from the bottles on my frame. I ate one energy bar between 30km and 60km and a gel at 70km. I had felt so full during most of the ride that I threw away my peanut butter sandwich somewhere around 50km. I was beginning to feel hungry, which is my preferred state to start a run anyway (not necessarily recommendable.) I passed the time check for the second stage, T2, dismounted my bike somewhat clumsily and ran with my bike towards the transition, only because everyone around me was running. I dropped my sunglasses again someone shouted at me and I retrieved them. I handed my bike to a marshal and proceeded to the transition tent to put on my runners. My face felt warm but a visit to the Portapotty indicated that I was well hydrated and ready for a half marathon. As I loped towards the first hill the loud-speaker boomed, "and our first Danish lady is running down the chute, Aarhus give her a large round of applause." She was done and I still had two and a half hours ahead of me. My legs felt fine, not wobbly, not fast but steady. I was closing in on my goal. It took me about 5km to start speeding up. I was not racing just pacing. After a while, I saw Anja. The course took us into the Old Town and then around three 7 km loops and then back out to the finish tent.

As you completed each loop you were given an elastic band to place around the wrist. First white, then red, then black. I had a new source of entertainment, now I could determine how far people were, how many loops they had completed. It was "fun" because the run was set up so that the loops often ran opposite each other. Faces became familiar, shops became familiar, even people dining in restaurants along the way became familiar.

I was so proud to be part of this group of athletes. I was under no illusion that I looked as tight and well-trained or even as young as most of them but there was no denying that I was one of them and it looked like I was going to finish Challenge Aarhus just like they were. I too had toiled in the pool, spent hours biking, pumped weights in the gym and had run on my own in the early morning. I belonged to this group of athletic people. I loved belonging to this group of athletic people. The horror of the early morning swim was slipping away and a warm feeling was taking over. The magic of participating in such a physically demanding event especially as a woman propelled me forward. I know I was not the only one feeling this because I could see the same magic in the eyes of the other female participants as we passed one another on the loops. We exchanged an almost imperceptible nod of respect. We ran through the Aros Museum three times, back and forth over bridges and even through underground car parks six times. As I approached the 17.8km marker I became emotional again, tears started running down my cheeks uncontrollably, I walked, I was getting so darn close. I walked but not much, I mainly ran at a comfortable, slow, steady pace. The temperature was rising and the water tables were positioned at every 2km. I drank a cup of water and a cup of energy drink at every station and doused myself with water. Only close to the end did I remember I was carrying my telephone, oh well hopefully it would survive. As I finished my third loop I turned out of the Old City onto the final stretch and then I heard "Mama, Mama, " they were there. Natasja, Tobias and Aleks ran with me, I noticed Tobias had a lose shoelace drifting in the wind, I told him to tie it I wasn't going to risk the last 500m. We came down the chute with them shouting, "You can do it Mama," it was overwhelming for some crazy reason I decided to sprint the last bit; I could hardly find enough oxygen in the air to fill my lungs. The loud speaker said, "here comes Tiffany Jolowicz from Great Britain," I felt like an Olympic athlete. I kept sprinting with Tobias and Natasja at my side, the clock showed 6.30 something. I crossed the line my chest tightened and the magnitude of my achievement and my family all crowded into my body, months of preparation could not ready me for this moment it was delicious. We had set ourselves this enormous, ridiculous target, we had trained, we had changed as people and we had overcome our fears. Whether we knew it or not there was no going back now. I went off to search for my t-shirt. Our times were:

	Me	Kirsten	Anja
Swim 1 km	0:22	0:20	0:21
Bike 90km	3:35	2:56	3:11
Run 21.1km	2:11	1:57	2:11
TOTAL	6:25	5:30	5:59

The t-shirt was a big disappointment but the rest was amazing. Recovery was quick much easier than the marathon of Madrid. I think this has to do with the swimming and biking disciplines preparing the body better for the run. We took the next few weeks off, relishing in our achievement and the fact that we did not have to train so much and often reliving our moment of glory. Back in Madrid, we set new goals, areas to improve on, we were setting ourselves up for our next challenge which we had not even determined but I don't think we even discussed whether there would be a second one it was just understood. One general goal was to improve the swimming experience. There was no way any of us was going to repeat the nerve-wracking performance of Aarhus. Even though I think I suffered the worst, none of us enjoyed a single moment of the Aarhus Bay washing machine. As it turned out my opportunity to settle my debt with the water came earlier than I had imagined.

GOLD: Use two swim caps, and put your goggles on between the two caps. Do this often as you practice at the pool, to practice how it feels. This prevents cap and goggle loss on the day.

SILVER: A friend sent me good luck wishes, "swim like a fish, run like a hare and bike as if you are wearing the yellow jersey." I kept repeating that all race day. By the way, fish have no arms, it is all core... The tip is to find your race day mantra, be on the look out for it in the last few days before the race.

BRONZE: Many professional and experienced athletes like to race at a certain "race weight." See Appendix B for (race) weight loss strategies. According to Rory Coleman of Marathon de Sable fame (look him up, interesting character,) to lose weight, you have to stop eating bread, pasta, rice etc. When he said this to us, we asked, " what about the carbs you need to train?" He replied, "You are wearing them." You have to be wise about this of course. We never really lost serious weight, much to our enormous disappointment.

BUITRAGO HALF-DISTANCE TRIATHLON 2012

7: Aqua phobia

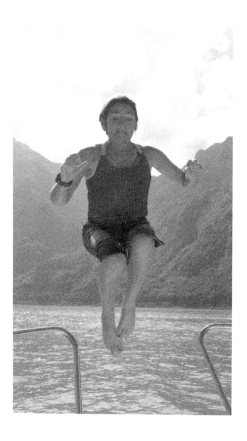

According to the Collins dictionary, aqua phobia is "an abnormal fear of water, especially because of the possibility of drowning"[7]

I am not sure if we feared drowning but there are many triathletes who have a great fear of water. The more I read about the swimming portion of the triathlon, the more I realised that my experience in Denmark was far from unique. Even at the full distance level, there is still a lot of fear for the swimming portion. See the comments from the Zürich Ironwomen in Chapter 24 More Aqua phobia.

Even though the swim is by far the shortest portion of the race it instils deep fears into full distance participants. Just looking at photos of the mass swim start of any long distance triathlon makes my heart beat faster.

The point about swimming is that it is not the hours spent in the pool sprinting back and forth or doing great distances that will change your swimming time or help with the panic and fears. The key to improving your swim experience is technique. This is good because although a challenge, it is not impossible to make yourself a better, more efficient, technically proficient, confident swimmer. A good swimming coach can literally change your life. In triathlon, "The swim seems to be a particularly dangerous time," said Andre La Gerche, a cardiologist at Melbourne's St Vincent's Hospital, triathlete and marathoner.[8]"Paradoxically, in the marathon, it's the opposite: it's the last mile of the event where the vast majority of fatalities occur." Researchers speculate that sprinting to the finish produces a rush of adrenalin that may trigger an abnormal rhythm in runners with susceptible hearts. In 'Fighting to Breathe' [9] la Gerche states that, "the swim leg of the triathlon, often held in open water, can be "extraordinarily stressful," he continues, "You have people climbing all over you.

Sometimes you're fighting to breathe, and that's not something the body is used to." Open-water racing triggers a clash of two mechanisms of the involuntary nervous system," according to researcher Mike Tipton, who runs the University of Portsmouth's Extreme Environments Laboratory. In a commentary for the British Journal of Sports Medicine in February 2013, he wrote "A fight or flight" response activated by physical exertion, cold water temperature or anxiety tries to speed up the heart rate and causes hyperventilation, just as the body is trying to slow the heart rate to conserve oxygen in response to facial wetting, water entering the mouth, nose and throat, and extended breath-holding," the scientist said. "Normally the two responses don't happen at the same time, but when they do, the heart can go into abnormal rhythms, which can cause sudden cardiac death." Nowadays, most swim starts are organised in pens, collecting swimmers with similar race prediction to start and finish more or less together. This makes for a much safer environment.

So the fears that we all face at the start line are more than psychological they are physical, based in our nervous systems. I wish I had known this before Aarhus. The key has to be understanding the fears and dealing with them and then employing good swim technique to gain confidence. Of course, not everyone suffers from this. Tatjana,

20, my second daughter is a great natural swimmer and we did our first race together which was an open water swim in the USA. She only prepared in an indoor pool, swam the distance a few times and said she was ready for the race. I tried to warn her about the potential for a panic attack, the washing machine effect, overcoming a fast heart rate at the beginning of the race, without trying to instil any fear in her that was not there. She cruised the race, finished in 1 hour and 6 minutes and when I asked her about how scary it had been she looked at me with a blank stare, she did not have any idea what I was talking about! Lucky her.

GOLD: Try this breathing exercise: See how few breaths you can take in a 3-minute period. Professional athletes can get as low as three. Sometimes it forces a type of panic and leads to greedily snatching breaths. This comes close to how I felt in the swim. Practice this and record your improvement. This is easily done in the car, on the train, bus, while waiting for someone. See: youtube.com/watch?v=S6BGyY7jTX0 or www.yogabasics.com/practice/dirga-pranayama/

SILVER: When you swim, swim intelligently, focussed and with precision. Better to swim 1000 metres of good stroke than 2000 metres sloppily. This is similar to wasted miles when running.

BRONZE: Read up about what constitutes good swim technique, watch videos and try to emulate the professionals.

8: Swimming across Lake Superior

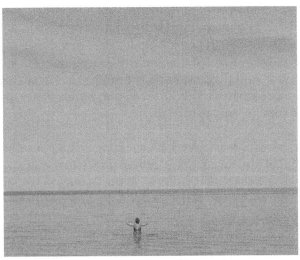

The Great Lake of Superior

July 2011

We lived for 13 years in Duluth, Minnesota. Four of the children were born there, so we feel a strong attachment to this beautiful part of the world and especially to Lake Superior. We try and return every summer to Madeline Island, one of the 22 Apostle Islands near Bayfield, Wisconsin. A few years back, I remembered a friend of ours' son swam the Point to La Pointe race. This is a 3.2 m swim race across Lake Superior, from the mainland town of Bayfield to the closest island, Madeline Island. Now that I was a triathlete, I was looking for different challenges. I looked up the Point to La Pointe swim.

"Swimming to the island has been a storied feat around the Bayfield area for decades. Point to La Pointe started as a community swim for 24 people in 2006. The event is now a race featuring more than 400 participants. Swimmers have encountered all of Lake Superior's moods over the years, from calm, flat water to strong crosswinds with 2-foot waves. The course follows the path of the winter "ice road", starting in Bayfield and landing at a beautiful family home on Madeline

Island. Spectators take the ferry across which offers views of the race. The fastest known time from shore to shore was set by Bryan Carlson, Edina, MN 43:24.5 in 2011."[10]

I could hardly resist the challenge but at the same time my head was haunted with the jellyfish and cold, waste-filled water of Denmark. I was certain I would feel better swimming in a lake versus salt water and I knew and loved the area. The water would be cold but unlikely to be 13.8ºC. It could be rough but it was a straight swim, no corners just a line of buoys to swim between with canoes on both sides protecting the entire course and hey all I had to do was swim, nothing was expected of me afterwards, just breakfast and I had seen the sweatshirts from previous years, they were awesome. I "took the plunge" and signed in.

Back to the pool. Kirsten and Maria were on vacation so I had to do some lengths on my own. I ran to the pool and swam the 3.2km distance one morning in early July, it was boring and lonely without them, but I did it, the furthest I had ever swum. Three days later, we left for the USA to attend a music camp at a University in Wisconsin, the same we had attended for many years. There, I rose each morning and ran a few km and then swam for 30 minutes in the afternoon, kind of tapering and preparing mentally, I was somewhat nervous. I figured I was fit enough to do the distance.

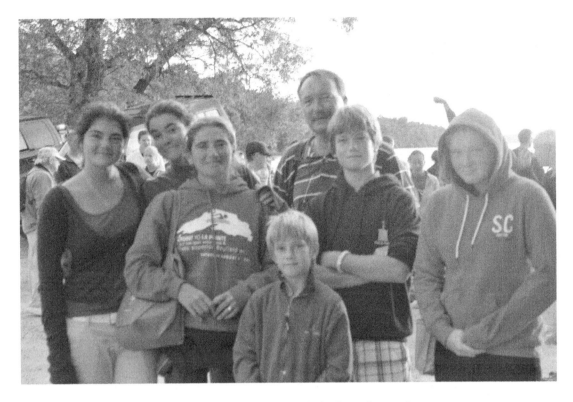

6:30 am on the mainland, before the swim

August 6th 2011

A week later the whole family rose at 6am to accompany me over to the mainland for the 7am start. They were becoming excellent supporters. All the swimmers waited for ages on the beach for 7am to roll around. The organizer, Scott read out the race rules at 6.45am finishing with "don't crowd each other, there is enough lake for all 369 of you." Lake Superior is the largest fresh water lake in terms of surface area in the world. Finally our wave came around. Wave is the name given to groups of swimmers starting at a certain time slot. Mike Tipton (previous chapter,) referred to wave as "pen." Typically all the women are in one wave. We advanced into the water and the gun went off. I waded in; it was quite warm and perfectly flat. So flat that the winner of the women's competition set a course record of 44.44 for the women, coming in 7th overall, behind a new general course record of 43.24 swum by Bryan Carlson again.

Conditions could not have been better. All I had to do was swim. I started off and within 20 seconds my heart rate seemed to have doubled and as the sand became distant and the water darkened, I panicked. My head started talking the negative again, "you have to swim like this for the next hour and a half; this is scary and stupid, get out." I nearly turned around. I stopped, started swimming some breaststroke and tried to control my breathing. I was so scared; I was losing control again. But I could not let myself beat myself, it would be just too easy to give in. I put my head into the water, this is my lake; this is the water I know so well. I started to try and find my stroke. Later I learned an excellent trick for this but at this stage it was just back and forth conversations with myself about continuing, not letting my head talk unless the conversation was positive, motivating and helpful. I kept going, at a breathtakingly slow pace. The next wave of swimmers started ploughing roughly and noisily past me. I ignored them. I found my stride and every 4 or 5 strokes orientated myself with the high group of trees Scott had pointed out to all of us at the start. "You can do this," I kept reminding myself. "You can swim well. " I let others pass, I found my own space and swam until I bumped into someone or they into me. I found a new space and kept going. I nearly ran into a rescue canoe about 6 times but I was basically going forward. At one point my head started thinking about all the fish in the water below me but I told it that the fish had for sure been scared away by this great body of thrashing swimmers. In Lake Superior there are some particularly gross eel type things called lampreys so I banished all thoughts and images of those immediately when they entered into my head. I swam further and then suddenly, I saw the half way buoy in front of me. Oh joy, I celebrated under water, congratulated myself on being such a strong personality, hard worker, I was beating my head, only half way to go.

Thoughts kept coming in unstructured sentences because my heart was beating so fast and there is no need to finish a sentence to yourself when you know what you mean. I tried to look at my watch to see how fast I was swimming. Disaster struck, the distance on my watch told me that I was only at the 300-metre buoy...what? How had that happened? I had been toiling for so long and only got so far? Not such a confident swimmer after all, very mediocre in the water now, still 2.9km to go. So far still? 116 lengths and probably another hour and 20 minutes. Full sentences now because somehow disappointment and negative thoughts form themselves perfectly. At least my battle was only with my head and not my heart rate. All I had to do was swim, settle down and swim. The dig deep moments of endurance sports. Just keep going. So I did, I had run out of options so all I had to do was swim, swim and swim some more. Some time later I reached the half way buoy. It was big, orange and beautiful! I touched it for good luck and carried on.

In my head whether biking, running or swimming I always think of the second half as downhill. I began to pull stronger I was going descending now. The mental tide was turning. I had never been in open water for this long in my life, I was so proud of myself, I was grinning under the water and was mesmerised by all the swimmers around me. It is very strange when really all you can see of hundreds of people in your general vicinity are arms, feet, swim caps and goggles. I was part of this group and so happy to be there. I soldiered on and on and on and on. The yellow arch marking the end of the course was growing. I could see people on the beach and every so often hear the loud speaker. I kept going, trying to concentrate on my stroke, on my technique trying to lengthen my body and arms, to stretch out towards the finish, grinning all the way. And suddenly I was there, the water became lighter I saw the sandy bottom, no jellyfish to accompany me in this time. My feet alighted on the red carpet in the bay and I stood up only to collapse. I came from horizontal to vertical too quickly and again a volunteer came to my rescue. She took me aside and de-velcroed the chip I had on my left ankle. I saw my whole family on the dock. It was 8:30am in the morning and I had achieved another dream! I walked up the red carpet beaming. I stripped off the top of my wetsuit because despite the cold water I had a warm face. Immediately Roland took a photo of me and I sent it to Kirsten with the message, "this time I beat the water," it felt so good, I was so proud of myself. The finisher's glory was becoming addictive; I began to relish this feeling of achievement. I had been scared, no denying it, but a tad less scared, I was beginning to build up a slightly more positive than negative attitude to open water swimming. I pulled on the fantastically cool red finisher's sweatshirt and we went back to the cabin. I took the rest of the summer off.

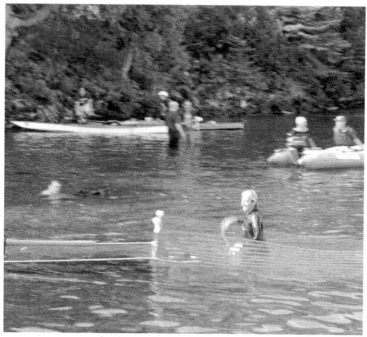
Arriving at Madeline Island.

Overcoming one's fears is one of the greatest gifts of triathlon. This is the mental battle. I used to hate flying, especially turbulence. Through swimming I learned to dig deep inside myself and use my brain as a helpful resource. I have since done some public speaking and am able to control my nerves and body much better. I have had a few MRI's, which I find horribly claustrophobic but am able to control the urge to panic. When training for a long distance race, a lot of the training is physical but a lot is mental too. The mental side, as discussed with rational and irrational motivators in Chapter 2, Obsessive. The mental aspect of long distance racing is both a powerful negative and positive force. The negative debate pulsing through the head sews seeds of doubt and lowers confidence. The positive forces enable you to push your body much further than you might imagine it can physically go. It is the mental side which forces you to train when physically you do not feel like it at all and it is the mental side which propels you on the day of the race and the mental side which relishes the victory.

GOLD: Engaging a swim teacher is a good idea. S/he will teach you how to swim and train properly so there are no wasted lengths in the pool. This has two benefits. Number one you will not emerge so exhausted from the swim portion and two you will learn to save leg energy, which is crucial for the next part of your triathlon day. A good technique will give you a good rhythm and that will help with stabilising your heart rate. Crucial is the bilateral breathing, which you really should master especially in the open water situation. Also you will need to learn to sight the buoys.

SILVER: Swimming at the pool can get boring and well into the training schedule it might become a chore. Going with someone helps. We used to split up the 1000metre stretches into 100metre challenges. I would determine what we did for 4 lengths and then Kirsten would determine the next four and so on. This kept our minds working because we always had to come up with a new challenge, no repetition. E.g. just arms with open fingers or fists, sprints, crawl legs and breaststroke arms. Anything we could think of to trick the mind into having a good time.

BRONZE: For sighting practice (which is teaching you to keep going in the right direction,) we would place a float or water bottle at the far end of the pool and look for it every 5 breaths. The smaller the sighting item, the better because it forced us to focus.

9: Real triathletes train, they don't work out

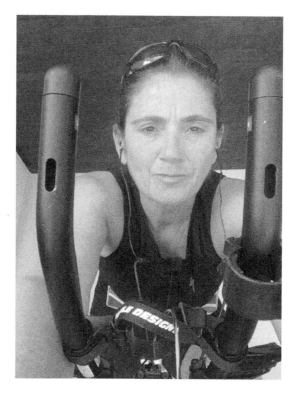

One of the 100's of bike turbo sessions

September 2011

We returned from the USA to Madrid late August and the kids began school. There was never any discussion as to whether we would do another half distance triathlon; we were addicted to the whole experience. I loved the camaraderie we had, the discussions about equipment and training schedules. I loved pushing my body and sweating hard. So much of our lives revolved around training and nutrition. We fell back into our old training routine. Once a week we met at school, ran 5km to the pool and swam. I did Pilates once a week. Kirsten spent more time at the gym doing weights and working on the machines. Given that the weather was unpredictable and to keep biking, the three of us started doing Spin classes with a new instructor, Sydney from Brazil. It was hard to follow his directions with the pounding music and his strong accent in Spanish, but he certainly had an inspiring six-pack. The only time I was ever ahead of Maria or Kirsten on the bike was when I took the front row in Spin! I enjoyed looking back at them. During the year we learned more about our bodies and started to track our heart rates on a more regular and informed basis. While Tobias was at basketball matches, I continued with the run sprints in a nearby park for 30 minutes as his team did their warm-up. At one point my heart rate was 205 beats per minute, but I think that was a technical error, either of my heart or the monitor.

We were building up for our second half distance and Maria's first, in Buitrago, a medieval village an hour north of Madrid. If you ever find yourself in Buitrago, it is also home to a tiny Picasso museum, housing the small, but worth-visiting collection of Picasso's barber, Eugenio Arias. Buitrago EcoTriMad half distance was to be our A Race of the season and it was to take place on 12 May 2012. Preparation for this was very different as we were able to get to know the territory better. Due to its proximity to home, we were able to bike the route four times before the race. This was hilly countryside, quite different to Aarhus, actually much tougher in many ways. The hills were substantially steeper, but the course was 14 km shorter. It was two loops of a 35km course, which meant that the trick when training was to keep going after the first loop. I hated that battle. It was always so hard because we passed the car and had to force ourselves to keep going. We biked both the Buitrago loop and the bike trail closer to home as our bike training. I never really enjoyed either.

Over the 9-month training period, we swam more critically and tried to improve our strokes. We bought swimming gadgets, like paddles, Kirsten even tried a waterproof iPod which she did not use much. The other gadgets were a good investment; they definitely helped us focus on our strokes and broke some of the boredom of swimming. We bought hand-shaped paddles from Zoggs and foam floats, which fit snugly between the legs for arms only and we used the same float held between our hands, arms stretched out, for leg only work.

Running we mainly did on our own. Sometimes Kirsten and Maria went out together over the weekends. I did not want to ruin their pace so I ran a lot on the treadmill, watching movies. Sometimes I would do back-to-back movie sessions, running for 3 ½ hours watching two movies. Later, I came to regard some of this as junk miles but sometimes whatever it takes to keep you training is more important than being efficient about the training. Maria started running with a super fit Dad from school and the two of them would run together for 3 hours, him talking all the way.

15 April 2012

As a B race challenge, we decided to run the Vienna marathon, decided, mainly because I have friends there and we thought we could stay at their house on the Saturday evening before. It turned out they were not at home that weekend but we had already registered. I had just returned from 10 days in Senegal where I had run about 5km in total, had done some yoga, lost 2kg (I was convinced it was all my well trained muscle just dropping off my bones.) Somewhat unprofessionally, 27 days before our A race, Buitrago, we were doing a B+ race. For some reason we considered that we should do a marathon as part of our training. This is definitely not necessary when training for a half distance tri. We would have preferred to do a marathon a little earlier in our schedules but Maria's 40th birthday party got in the way so Vienna was our best option. The Saturday morning before the race I woke up with a mild fever and a huge cold, I had basically lost my voice, but the tickets were booked the t-shirts paid for (extra €20,) and we had to go. We arrived in Vienna at 7:30pm on the Saturday evening before the marathon and grabbed a cab. The taxi driver asked why we were in Vienna and we told him to run the marathon, "I thought so," he replied, I thought for the first time that just maybe I looked like an athlete! Finally, we sat down to a pasta dinner around 9pm, which was way too late. We arrived at the hotel and the receptionist gave us our race packets, which my friend had picked up the afternoon before and dropped off at the hotel for us. The t-shirt was definitely not worth it. I think I have since given it away, the only marathon shirt I have ever parted with. We went to bed soon after and I tried really hard all night not to cough and sneeze and sniff and snore. We awoke around 5:30am and showered. It is at those moments you just think how dumb these endurance sports are. Why does one put oneself through this scary experience? What is it that drives one to take this challenge? These emotions came back and nearly ravaged me in Zürich a year later. It reminded me of this quote I read somewhere,
"A man must love a thing very much if he not only practices it without any hope of fame and money, but even practices it without any hope of doing it well." G. K. Chesterton.

In the breakfast room at 6:30am, there were hundreds of fit looking people tucking into coffee and muesli, bananas and bagels. Voices were kept low but everyone had a sort of smug little grin. We all felt excited, nervous and privileged I suspect. Ultimately it is a privilege to be able to participate in this game. Firstly to be healthy enough to submit your body to the rigours of training, secondly mentally fit enough to be able to submit your mind to the rigours of training and finally to have the family, time and resources to dedicate oneself to the rigours of training!

This small piece from an article by Gary Robbins is a reminder of this: "I met one of Canada's most experienced adventure racers at the time and I was asking him for some training tips," he responded with, "Training? I've never trained a day in my life." "Excuse me?" "I play everyday, but I never go out to train. I go outside to play in the woods and to interact with nature. When I stop enjoying it like play, then it becomes work. Work, no matter what form it may take, will always feel like work." http://garyrobbins.blogspot.com.es/2013/11/finding-motivation.html

Similarly as Gerry Duffy explains in his excellent book, "Tick, Tock, Ten" about his completion of ten full distance triathlons in ten consecutive days, otherwise known as a Deca Iron Triathlon, "I do this because I can."

We packed our bags, stored them downstairs, went to the bathroom for the 14th time that morning and left the hotel at 7.15am. The race did not begin until 9am, but we were not going to sleep anyway. The hotel was 1.5km from the start so we walked along the tramline with many others going in the same direction. We visited the bathroom another four times; Vienna was special for us because it had a tent just for ladies' toilets. So much cleaner, the line was more civil and there was even toilet paper and hand cleaner.

My father died in 1982 at the age of 46, he led a pretty sedentary life as a stockbroker, did not smoke, did not drink excessively but had high cholesterol. I too have high cholesterol but keep it under control by fitness. He used to play the clarinet not well, I can not really remember how well but his favourite all time piece was Mozart's Clarinet Concerto in A major. We played it at his funeral. This being Austria, instead of playing loud pop songs over the speaker system in the hour or so before the race they were playing classical music. As we proceeded to the line-up, on came Mozart's Clarinet Concerto. For me starting any of these endurance races is an emotional experience, I suppose it has to do with the mental preparation and all the hormones racing around. Couple that with Mozart's Clarinet Concerto and I buckled, tears rolled down my cheeks. It was sad and beautiful at the same time; I wished he had been here watching me.

9:00am, we were off, Garmin watches buzzed all around us as we stepped over the timing mat. Kirsten and Maria disappeared into the blur of bodies. I kept a good pace completing 10km in 52 minutes, which I held until the half marathon. There were water tables every 5km and in some cases every 2km. The Madrid marathon has water tables every 5km so I assumed this was standard practice at every marathon. My marathon plan has always been to run 5km and walk through each water table drinking a cup of water and a cup of energy drink. Thus I always break my marathon up in 8 bite size chunks. The higher number of water tables in the first half of the race confused me and shook my rhythm as I was not sure what the distribution would be at later stages of the race; this cost me time. Note to self "study the course map before the race and come up with a hydration plan."

The most pleasurable part of the marathon was the last 300 metres. They had placed the large blue motorway markers that one sees as one is approaching a motorway exit in the car except here they were indicating the last 300, 200 and 100 metres to the finish line.[11] It felt like someone organising the race had a sense of humour, it made my finishing smile even broader.

I still picture these signs often when I am doing sprinting practice or finishing another long distance run. I can still visualise that finish and I deliberately recapture and enjoy again that delicious, warm feeling of deep contentment as I was approaching the Vienna finish. It goes so far that when driving sometimes I find myself smiling at those signs on the road. That is the crazy and useful visualisation technique of a distance athlete.

All of us had hoped to do a personal best in Vienna. We had hoped that dropping to 171metres above sea level versus 600metres above sea level in Madrid would give us an advantage. Have no idea if that is a reasonable thought or not, but it sounded quite professional to us to think that thought. We imagined that we must be in better shape than ever and that our enthusiasm for this would serve us well. In the end none of us was particularly pleased with our time. For some reason our legs were not carrying us swiftly, maybe the extra training had tired us more. Unexpectedly, all three of us took more than 13 minutes to complete the last 2.2km. Final times you see below. Maria the same as Madrid a year earlier, Kirsten 5 minutes slower and me 3 minutes slower, it did not make much sense, but hey you just never know.

Maria	3:22
Kirsten	3:44
Me	4:01

We learned that each marathon is different. This one we should have taken more warm clothes with us, especially for the end. Kirsten got very cold on completion. She was almost disorientated so we wolfed down the most delicious Bratwurst I have ever had in my life, it was at least 30cm long, thickly spread with the perfect combination of Ketchup and Mustard. Nicely stuffed, we went in search of some coffee to warm Kirsten from the inside out. I now know that a cup of coffee (especially for Kirsten) will reinvigorate in minutes. This marathon had fancy potties at the start but no pacing balloons. We talked about what had made this marathon perhaps not quite the success we had expected. We concluded first (and somewhat obviously) how important it is to read the race information and familiarise yourself with the course and its idiosyncrasies. Also somewhat obviously, we decided that you should eat your pre-race pasta at 6:30 pm the previous day so that you are hungrier for breakfast and then not hungry at the start line like we were. Remain flexible, think on your feet as it were, if the water tables are not as expected you have to go with the flow, if you are hungry eat a gel earlier than you might have planned and take what is available. This worked for and against me later in the IRONMAN Switzerland. Whatever, we had had a fun 24 hours and I just loved running and being with my wonderful friends. We had had another new experience and learned more about endurance sports and ourselves.

GOLD: Learn about the technique of visualisation as a mental tool. Start practicing it on your runs, swims and bike rides.

SILVER: Develop a visualisation library, using the events (marathons, swims etc.) you complete as part of your visualization library. Add certain places from your training repertoire to this library. I often use a 400-metre outdoor athletics track we used to train on in Spain when on my treadmill to push myself through a turbo running session. I picture myself running around this track, passing the pole-vaulters, the high jumpers, the sprinters warming up and the spectator stands. I became so good at this technique that when on a long solo bike ride I could reduce myself to tears visualising myself crossing the IRONMAN Switzerland finish line.

BRONZE: Study the course map before the race and come up with a hydration and nutrition plan.

10: Fighting dehydration at the Buitrago Half Triathlon

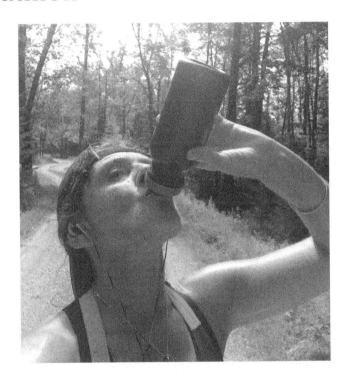

4 May 2012

One week out from Buitrago, we drove the hour north to look at the swimming location. We took a swimming pool temperature monitor with us. The shallow water measured 6ºC.

We emailed Joaquim, the Buitrago organiser, and he said according to them the water was 17ºC; this huge body of water was 7ºC warmer than the local outdoor swimming pool? We were a little sceptical to say the least. Anyway he said that on the day if the water were less than 13º C they would change the rules of the race.

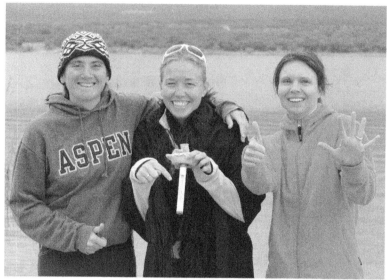
Testing the waters in Buitrago

We decided not to get in the water and instead went to ride the circuit. This was a hard ride; don't know why it just felt like a fight the whole way round. Maybe my legs were nervous or still tired from the marathon, but it seemed so much harder than the same ride we had done just before Christmas. Four months on, four months of training further and I felt worse, it just did not seem fair. Oh well bad dress rehearsal, good performance right? I was talking to myself, I had a lot of work to do, I had to get my head sorted out and my energy levels up. We finished the ride I was starving, I felt low, I only wanted to do one loop, I could not be bothered to fight the fight for a second loop. I forced myself to look forward to trying on the wetsuit again in the pool on Monday.

A week later, on Friday 11th we drove up to Buitrago to pick up our race packets and to see if we could have a quick dip in the water. Kirsten felt really sick so we did not swim. Things were not looking so good for Kirsten but apparently the outlook for the swim looked better as the temperature was pleasant enough, so the swim was on. We visited the finishing area, which was still being set up and cast a nervous glance at the hills. We drove home in silence, Kirsten concentrating on not throwing up and I concentrating on not panicking.

12 May 2012

Buitrago, officially, the EcoTriMad half distance tri race began at noon. It is hard to control one's nerves for so long and also hard to know what and when to eat. I ate a big sandwich at 4pm the day before and pasta at 5:30pm and then breakfast at 8am ish, followed by half a bagel and a banana at 11am.

We had arrived Saturday morning around 9:15am and started sorting out all our gear. For some reason, I seemed to have four times as much as everyone else. I dragged my stuff, which was in various bags, to the check-in line. I kept dropping water bottles and then my helmet and then my huge bike pump and looked like the total amateur I was. I even let go of my bike at one point and it clattered to the ground. It was just that my hands were shaking so much. Our bike brakes were checked and we were cleared into the boxes area. Yesterday this had been a mess of bike racks and blue tarpaulin, now it was organised and professional looking. 500 people had signed up for this, a small number of elites but mainly age-grouper men and a handful of courageous women. There were some familiar faces from our local gym, mainly the personal trainers and one or two other guys I recognised from spin class.

I went in search of the bathroom. They were located in a clean facility next to some showers and changing room, behind some trees of to the right of the lake. This visit was the first of maybe five visits before we started two hours later. I ended up around the back where they were dope testing, how cool were we participating in a sporting event where they have to dope test? I felt elite and sick all at the same time.

We hung around and around. Kirsten tried to do some yoga breathing, Maria stretched and I just lay half in the sun, half in the shade, trying to remember why we were here and why we were doing this. I kept trying to drag myself back to the moment, trying to focus on the finish line, la Meta. It was hot.

At 11.15am, we pulled on our wetsuits and headed down to the water. Somewhat distracted by the enormity of our undertaking, Anja walked off towards the beach, wearing her biking sunglasses, thinking she had her swim goggles on. I noticed this and she took them off, ran to her bike, where she had left her goggles neatly next to her helmet. She hurriedly placed her biking glasses where they belonged and clamped her goggles to her head, where they belonged. It was all just so nerve wracking. Minor details can change an entire race and this demonstrated the power of being in a team. More proof that triathlon is not an individual event for sure, well at the age-grouper level for anyway.

We donned our pink swim caps and huddled with the other female age-groupers, we were 21 in all. No one spoke much; we gingerly exchanged proud grins, again that look of athletic respect. We moved closer to the water's edge as the elite guys started, followed quickly by the elite girls. And before we knew it, at exactly 12:05pm, we were off. Oh god so scary, into the water, my heart pounding. I could not find my rhythm. I tried to get my 3 stroke breathing going it was elusive, my heart was trying to "break out of my body and fly away, like a bat out of hell," the song kept going around and around in my crazy head, now I knew what Meatloaf was talking about: triathlon swimming. 30metres in, maybe three minutes I don't know, I was ready to quit. I felt myself swim to the left to escape the madness. Then the head conversation began, 7 hours of this; give into this panic after all the preparation of the last few years. Where was my iron will? I just wanted out, I looked around for the rescue rafts there was one quite close, I could either swim to the raft or try to get to the next buoy. I spotted a rescue raft at the next buoy, so I did a deal with myself; get to the next buoy and then decide. I worked my way back into the frenzy and started on a two stroke breathing rhythm when I could, followed by breaststroke when my head could not take being in the water. Somehow, I made it to my target buoy, which must have been about 500 metres into the race. Note to self; have a clear idea of the distances between the buoys. It was madness, frigging madness, how had I let myself been drawn into this madness again?

OK 1.4km to go. I turned located the next buoy and started my 3-stroke-1-breath rhythm. This was familiar even if the surroundings were horribly alien. I kept looking up and around. I saw green and blue caps from the hundreds of male age-groupers. No one swam over me in this washing machine and I was pushing forward with each stroke. I made it to the third buoy and around it and then my left calf muscle cramped. I had never had this before although I had read about others suffering from this. I stretched my muscle as best I could whilst trying to keep moving and pulling myself forward. I told myself I was half way round although I was not sure about this, lying to one-self is an interesting triathlon phenomenon. Following my positive train of thought, mind over matter, given I was so far I permitted myself to I relax a little, this I hoped would relieve the tension in my leg. I allowed myself the luxury of thinking that I could complete this race. I forced myself to be present in the moment, which is both scary and important in the water. I decided to focus on everything in my immediate vicinity, firstly my body, my breathing, my stroke, the guy ahead. How could I improve my stroke and my swim? Suddenly I was in charge for the first time in the water. I could think more clearly. I could think, not just ramble or waste energy on stopping certain thoughts. I was able to have rationale, constructive thoughts. It dawned on me that instead of fearing the guy ahead, I should just follow his foot bubbles and probably I would be going in the right direction. I tried to draft but was still way too nervous to succeed at that. I steered well away from him and well away from a higher heart rate. I had been over-ambitious in my newfound confidence, whoops! I was in control but the humbling nature of triathlon made sure that I realised that I could lose that control very quickly if my heart rate climbed. I felt good because I was sure I was up with the front women, somehow, I was positioned right on the inside so was not even able to drift off to the shoreline like I had done in Aarhus. I almost began to feel comfortable. As we rounded the fourth buoy my left calf cramped up again. I pulled with my arms letting my legs just dangle, trailing behind I tried to stretch the muscle, all the time rebuking it for letting me down. I still needed my left leg. It still had work to do! Only 500metres left; how often had I done 20 lengths in the pool? I started to swim a little faster, I did not really want my heart rate to increase too much because I knew that panic was only a heart beat away but I accelerated because I felt invigorated. The beach was coming closer and that was all that mattered. I was sure I had come in in the first wave of women; that was how confident I felt now. I thought I was among the elite women! Haha. As I exited the water I started to peel off my wetsuit, someone shouted my name. I love seeing people I know on the course. Who knew me here? It was Deb, a mother from school; I recognised her voice. As I ran up the ramp out of the water, I saw Deb and her two kids. She said the others had just come through. Huh, I thought I was well ahead of them, hadn't I just come in with the elite women? Hey I thought oh well at least I did not have to swim again. I ran to T1 and saw Kirsten and Anja who were just departing on their bikes, "good swim guys," I managed to shout as they disappeared. It was easy to find my bike because most of the ladies were through by then, not sure whom I thought I was swimming next to in the water. Off I went downhill and then uphill. My heart was pounding again, my legs were tired and I had to focus. 3.5km small incline. There were many people around me, overtaking but I doggedly stuck to my task, ate a gel, drank some energy drink and thanked God I had survived the swim and then I started talking to my quadriceps.

The 75km was long and it would take me 3.5hours, I was definitely not a biker yet. Note to self; grow some quads. The ride was twice 35km loop and then the 2.5km back to Transition. As I finished the first loop, the leader, followed by a motorbike overtook me at lightening speed. His time, ablaze above the courtesy vehicle in front of him, was 2 hours and 18 seconds, he turned left heading for T2. As he rushed by, followed by me for a few brief seconds, someone shouted, "there's the first woman," victor's glory for about three seconds, then I turned right, giving away my status as slow woman and started my second loop. At the 35km water station they had run out of water. This was located at the top of a hill and I was looking forward to stopping and guzzling water. I did not need a banana, or a gel or an energy drink I just wanted nothing else but water. It was a hot, hot day; the temperature was a good 31ºC and rising. I had two bottles on my bike with a 50:50 PowerAde-water mix, at least that is what I thought I had. We were in the mountains at 1200 metres above sea level and I was drying out, I could feel it. There was another water station 20km from this one in a small village. I focused on their bountiful supply of water. Suddenly Kirsten came out of the crowd, she had thrown up countless times and had decided to quit. "Come on," I told her, "you are a biker, you can do one more loop." A voice from the crowd said, "she looks much better now than she did ten minutes ago." I moved on and then seconds later I recognised her behind me. We cycled up the first hill together. We have never cycled up a hill together; a sure sign that her body was not performing at top capacity. Eventually she dug deep and off she went.

I was back to my solo conversation, my baking tongue and salt-crusted red face. Shortly after, her stomach cramps and some kind of virus got the best of her and she dropped out, it took her body a week to recover. Dehydrating and desperately, I groped for my second water bottle; it was water! I remember it standing on the kitchen counter and I had hated to throw away water to replace it with PowerAde so I left it as just water. I rationed myself for 20km up and down and through the hills. Unbelievably the next water station too had run out of water. I could see three guys ahead, I passed them and we kept in a loose group for the whole loop. With 20km to go they were out of water too. I was in trouble, I was dehydrating, I was very hot, my legs were tired and I was beginning to obsess about water. I caught up with a guy who was very hot. At one point he screamed in pain and stopped. I never saw him again. At the base of the mountain I passed another guy sitting by the road, "estas bien?" "Si, no te preoccupes." He quit too. My mouth was burning and my tongue felt like the arid African soil, I pictured a photo I had taken in Senegal that was how my tongue felt. I was trying desperately hard to distract my mind from the discomfort of dehydration by entertaining myself with whatever images I could pull up. I focused on a plan, if I wanted to complete a half marathon I had to re-hydrate at T2. I drank some more energy drink, which felt like drinking seawater and pushed on. This was familiar territory because we had cycled the course four times before the race. I formulated a plan, somewhat late in the day I coined my mantra for the race, "The plan: I had to finish by 7pm," it was now 4:05pm by the time I got to T2 I was going to get out of my

80

bike gear, take a cold shower in the changing facilities and grab as much water as I could. I had read that one of the most efficient ways to reduce body temperature is to cool down the skin. A cold shower was exactly what the doctor was ordering. I topped the hill, flew down the remaining 2km downhill and turned into the familiar transition area.

I was in luck Anja's family, Kirsten and Maria were in T2. Maria had quit the race in the very early stages of the swim. This was a shock for all of us since she had already finished a full distance triathlon. It just proves that each race is different and there is no room for complacency at any stage of the race. In her words, "The race was over within 5 minutes. Many people had expectations and I think I got nervous. My heart started to beat way too fast from the start of the swim, from fear. I also think that I started out way too fast. I think what I did wrong was that someone had said that you should swim on your back and relax if you were stressed. But that was just harder and it just made everything worse. So the lesson learned is; if you don't know how you react in the water go very slowly in the beginning, as it is hard to get the heart rate down once it has gone up. AND if your heart rate goes up just swim very slowly to the side where people aren't passing over and around you. Try to just float and think positive thoughts and then start slowly to swim again."

I ran around to get my bike parked and told them I needed water. I drank 2 litres straight and grabbed two more bottles to douse over my over-heating body and started off on the run, well walk because after all that water I had a stitch! "I had to finish by 7pm." Everything felt urgent now so that was why I guzzled. Note to self: sip don't guzzle. At least given I had so much water I had not had to waste time taking a shower. After 2km I ran through the wood at the furthest point of the run and with 19km to go, I fell and started crying. Lying on the ground with a bleeding knee and elbow, I picked myself up. I still had a stitch and I still had a lot to do. It took me 7km to rebalance my hydration and ditch the stitch. Around that time I started running with a guy with horrible back pain. We managed 4km together. I had found a kind of rhythm. I walked the up-hills and ran the down, there did not seem to be much flat ground. It was a dirt track so footing was tricky. As I came into the medieval town of Buitrago for the second time, I saw Natasja, then Tobias then Maria, Klaus and Aleks and Klara. The two of them were carrying a sign said, "Run as if you have stolen something!" I couldn't but I kept going. As I left the town behind to complete the last loop it began to hail, thunder and lightening. It hurt on my back, which I later realised had become quite burned despite the factor 45 I put on at 11.30am. I had three guys running behind me, from a starting field of 500. I hoped they finished by 7pm. I had seen that Anja and Gadi were ahead of me as we passed on the loops. I was closing in on the "meta." It felt good. My endurance was there and I still had 20 minutes in hand. I could see the time on the huge village clock sticking out above the roofs of Buitrago. I was going to finish. As I ran past the medieval walls of the fortress, marking the last 500 metres Tobias by my side I could not believe it. I ran into the courtyard of the 15th century fort, 6 hours and 50 minutes after I started. Those still around applauded and cheered as I ran over the finish line with 3 of my kids. In the photo, you cannot see Aleks, he is right behind me. As my husband reached down to give me a congratulatory kiss I said, "that was hard work, not sure this body has a full distance tri in it!" Little did either of us know. Roland would disagree he says he did know!

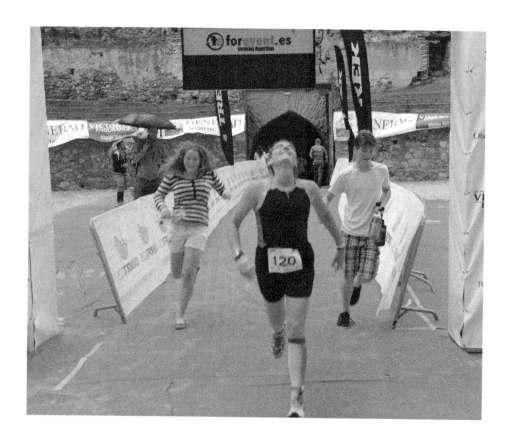

Approximately 500 people started that race and 389 finished I came in 384th. 22% dropped out.

Swim	0:43
Bike	3:27
Run	2:30
TOTAL	6:55

GOLD: You just never ever know how the day will turn out, but most important, don't push yourself too far, keep going but always be safe.

SILVER: A repeat but I think it is important to recognize the impact of a mantra. Let it flow, breathe, find your mantra even in the toughest of situations. Quoting Gerry Duffy, the total nut who completed ten full distance triathlons in ten days, again from his book," Tick Tock Ten," he survived by counting backwards, e.g. 180 to bike, 179, 178 etc., 41 km to run 40 km to run through to 3 km to run 2, 1 and each km he celebrated! It is a book well worth reading.

BRONZE: It doesn't matter if you come in nearly last, finishing is still an awesome achievement. Because as John Bingham said "The miracle is not that I finished, it is that I had the courage to start."

11: We may be losers but we are not quitters, turning failure into success.

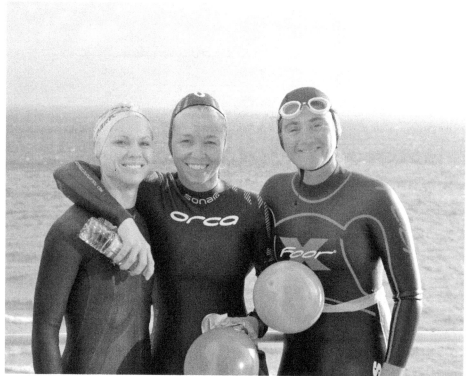

Testing the waters in Buelna

Maria's experience in Buitrago convinced us that we needed some help with the swim, so a decision was made that we needed proper swimming lessons. Three weeks later we found ourselves at the gym again, this time poolside. This must have been my first swimming lesson in 35 years. It was awesome, an Epiphany. I have always admired those who seem to glide effortlessly, almost above the water. I finally had my first taste of it. The perfect stroke requires long reaches, the longest reaches you can imagine and a good turn of the shoulders during the breath. The more you turn without rolling, the further the front hand is reaching, the more the distance you cover before it enters the water. This long reach also allows for a nice long breath. Secondly, the concentration on the long stroke reduces the heart rate giving a greater sense of control. Greater speed does not come from ploughing through the water with a quicker stroke; it is about technique. This all keeps the heart rate where it should be when panic rears its ugly head. We finally got the impression that we would be able to respond to that panic by slowing our breathing and slowing the momentum of the heartbeat, by simply slowing down our stroke; it was so exciting.

The sting of not finishing Buitrago was too much for my triathlon buddies to bear. They were annoyed with themselves and they wanted to test their fitness at the half-tri distance again. Thus, the inevitable happened, burning with not having completed Buitrago, they dived into the Internet in search of another half distance triathlon. They were looking for a race close to Madrid, still with some open registrations and within the next month. Maria found one in Buelna. The only problem was that it is located at the northern tip of Spain, on the ocean no less, the Cantabrian Sea if you wish to down-tone the waves and wind patterns from ocean to sea. Kirsten was not convinced and proposed Valladolid, same date, two hours closer and a river swim, factory waste yes, but no waves. Not quite sure how, but Maria prevailed, Kirsten caved and they signed up for Buelna. The focus on the swimming became sharper. We began to take our pool sessions very seriously. We improved, but how would we feel this in the real water? To assuage Kirsten's sea fears and to see Comilla's Cove, site of the Buelna swim, for ourselves; a trip was planned. We drove the 430km north. The beach was gorgeous, the hotel perfect. We went out for dinner and set our alarms for 7.30am. We awoke. The sea was calm. We pulled on our wetsuits and looked out again, in three minutes the sea had become a torrid, angry battlefield. The wind was gusty, from the North East, which meant waves were lashing the beach. What had happened to our perfect confidence-building swim? We exited the hotel, descended the steep steps and onto the beach.

As we walked across the beach, it was like we had walked into a desert storm. We had to pull on our goggles to protect our eyes and Maria's beach board and safety balloons kept hitting me. We went to the farthest end of the cove, seeking refuge from the wind behind the tiny harbour wall. We figured we should swim with the current because it seemed way too strong to fight. We got into the water; it was about 17ºC. We pulled our balloons onto our backs and started to swim gingerly. Kirsten was resisting putting her head into the water. We told her she had to, no option. We went with the current for a while and then decided to swim out. Then the strangest thing happened. We felt comfortable. Despite the moving water, we were able to glide above. Our new stroke techniques were giving us space to breath, think and stretch. It was nothing short of amazing. Suddenly we felt alive and happy in the water, not like fish happy but happy. We felt stronger than ever, all three of us. We went back and forth a few times, we breathed on the non-wavy side, every two strokes and felt ourselves pulling efficiently and unhurriedly through the water. As we stopped to take stock of this momentous tri-moment we were full of excitement. We all grabbed onto Maria`s beach board, bobbing up and down in the swollen waves. We high-fived and felt really good. They say triathlon is about overcoming fears; we were on our way. Kirsten and Maria knew now that they could do the challenge. Later we took the car and more or less drove the 90km cycle route, which contained some tight bends and long up-hills. But my friends buoyed by their swimming experience did not see them as too much of a problem now!!

7 July 2012

Triatlon Valle de Buelna. These are Maria's words on recalling the day:

"Here the race started at 1pm which was convenient from "not having to get up early in the morning" perspective, but it was hot and the water was wavy, not calm like in the mornings. The swimming was in the open sea, so coming a few days before and preparing was nice. I got my confidence in the water back again. The women started first which meant that on the second lap the men were swimming their first lap beside me. Kirsten and I swam to the side and no men swam over us. It was reassuring that Kirsten and I had decided to swim together at this smaller race. I felt confident having her there. At the Zürich race that would have been impossible because there were just too many people all around you. Doing the loop 10 times running was BORING and not too much fun."

They called me on completion, their voices sounded like bubbly 7 year olds, they were so happy, they had crossed the line together, holding their kids' hands as they would a year later in Zürich.

	MARIA	KIRSTEN
Swim	0.47	0.47
Bike	3.16	3.08
Run	1.49	1.57
TOTAL	6.00.06	6.00.06

GOLD: If you want something enough it can be yours. Channel your anger and indignation or fear of failure into something positive.

SILVER: Learn from a DNF- Did Not Finish... "That which does not kill us, makes us stronger" - Friedrich Nietzsche

BRONZE: Triathlon is not only an individual sport; it is also very much a team sport. If you put your IRONMAN, whichever one you did, on your CV you may get the response that it is all about the individual. It can be important to remind employers that this is not the case.

IRONMAN SWITZERLAND
JULY 2013

12: To the world they are my family, to me; they are the world.

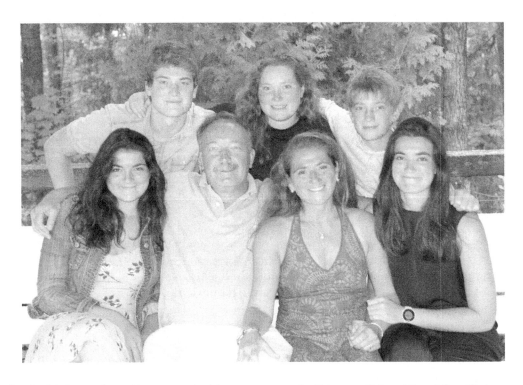

I don't think an ultra distance triathlon or even a half is possible without familial support, whether you are 21 or 61. The comments from my tri-sisters at Zürich show that behind every successful triathlete woman, there is an incredible group of people. See their comments in Chapter 25, "It is amazing how far you can go if someone believes in you."

Whilst Kirsten and Maria were my tri-team, my family was my everything-else-backup. Here is our team the day before IRONMAN Switzerland.

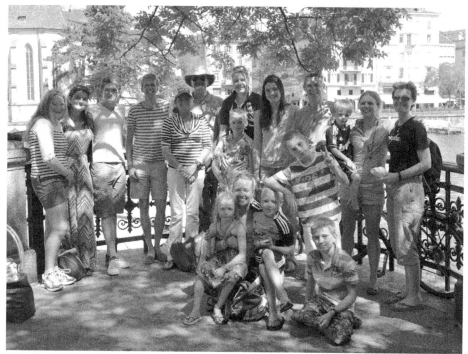

Natasja, Tatjana, Tobias, Klaus, me, Roland, Emil, Lars, Sacha, Ian, Karl-Oscar, Maria, Chloë, Klara, Kirsten, Jeppe & Aleks

My family members encouraged, they listened, they took the journey with me. Roland drove me to half marathons and marathons at the crack of dawn. He took care of the kids. My birthday and Christmas presents nearly all had a triathlon theme, from Garmin watches to a Training Diary. My mother bought me IRONMAN-brand socks, my brother, biking gloves, my sister and brother-in-law countless useful accessories, which I did not even know existed. My life became a tri-fest and I was loving it. My family knew to give me space if I hadn't trained or when I had a big smile they knew that was the cue to ask how far I had run or biked. Most people around me knew I was involved in this crazy sport. Tatjana's basketball team even asked me to train them to improve their fitness and we ran a 6 km Carrera de la Mujer, a run just for women, together in Madrid.

The enormity of a full distance triathlon brought out an emotional side to me, which I had never really associated with sport. Maybe this is part of the difference between ironmen and ironwomen, am not sure. Reading the comments in Chapter 25 always brings tears to my eyes.

The ultra triathlon distance goal is not only about the athlete. Family members invest too in the endeavour and cannot help but be touched by the energy and magic of endurance triathlon. That's what I thought but of course there is another side of the story. I asked Roland to share some of his tips for the partner of an ironwoman, in his words: He titled his document, "Triathlete Spousal Abuse."

"Spouse's/partner's tips to living with a triathlete:

1) Understand what she is getting into
-Realise and embrace that once the triathlon bug has taken root, priorities will change.
-Preparing for triathlon is a way of life.
-Be prepared and support a rigorous training schedule that will take her away from the home environment for many hours every week
-Be open to a new circle of friends based around triathlon and talking and discussion topics will drift towards triathlons, the training needed, what foods should be eaten, hydration, sleep etc. etc.
-Be prepared for and don't question immense spending on the kits for the different sports (especially the biking)

2) Stay true to yourself
-Although you support, don't let yourself be talked into their life style unless you want to become a triathlete yourself
-You will be encouraged to join in and if you are not careful you will find yourself with an expensive racing bike you know you will only use infrequently and then discard
-You will notice that the meals you are presented will also change (definitely healthier), just make sure that there is a clear understanding that you are not preparing for a triathlon
-Avoid mixing your exercise schedule up with that of a triathlete otherwise you end up doing things that don't inspire you (like working on your inner self/core) and will destroy your enjoyment of exercise.
-You will also learn the true meaning of divine discontent, as nothing will ever be good enough.

3) Prepare well in advance for the actual race.
-A triathlon can take more than 15 hours and if you have children in tow you will need to know how to keep them energised and excited during the different stages
-Book appropriate accommodation early so that you have a comfortable base from which to leave and come back to during and after the event
-Make sure that you have suitable transportation set up to get you to the different stages, for the whole family and potentially a bike etc.
-Take enough food and drinks along to keep everybody happy
-The swim is the least inter-active for the spectator. Once they are off you will only see a lot of splashing and will soon not be able to identify your triathlete.
-Best to let the kids rest for the long day ahead
-The biking is more entertaining but also fast paced. Your partner will love seeing you, family and friends along the way and will usually spend a few minutes with you to recover and replenish.
-So best to position yourself close to a break area.
-Make sure you have a good idea of where on the bike route they are. We once spent an hour expecting her to come by when she had already passed the location beforehand.
-The running at the end is probably the best place to support your partner. Often the run will pass the same point two or more times, so you can position yourself along the route and see them come around.
-NEVER miss the finish. This is the ultimate moment of triumph after months of hard work and not being there will not go down well. If you have children they can often run the last 50 meters with your partner, which is highly appreciated and allows you to take the victory picture.

4) Recognise the emotional impact of a triathlon
-The triathlon will be a very emotional event for your partner as she will fight with herself to control fears (for example in the tumble drier), push through ups and downs and be emotionally overcome by what she has achieved.
-Small gestures are incredibly powerful A gift that can be worn during the race and presented the evening before during diner (we bought a gold infinity chain before the Zurich triathlon.)
-Having the whole family hiding in the car at 5.30am in the morning when she only expected you to bring her to the start.
-Having the children run the last 50 meters wish your partner.
-A kiss at the end however sweaty your partner is.

5) Finally make sure that you also have fun during the event.

-Plan it as a family outing and try and get the most out of the location where the event is taking place."

Beth our friend and yoga teacher wrote a thesis on yoga and its benefits for long distance athletes. Using Kirsten, Maria and me as her guinea pigs, she developed a yoga practice for our unique aches and stiffnesses. She took a holistic view of our training, including helping with nutrition. To gain an overview of the impact that our training was having on those around us, she asked our family members to write something about their impressions of the full distance tri training on their lives; this is what my daughters wrote:

Sacha:
"My mom as a triathlete is a huge inspiration in so many ways, but here is just a list of random thoughts that I hope can help you out ☺

1.   Perseverance: everyday that she gets up and runs/ bikes/ swims/ does Yoga/ Pilates/ random fitness training is a testament to her character. I know she does not always want to do this, but the fact that she does shows us how you just have to keep going. I think we all keep this in our minds when studying for exams, writing essays, working on presentations, practicing instruments, anything really. She shows us how if you keep going at it you can succeed.

2.   Keeping Fit: hearing her talk about how to eat right, what muscles to train and how to build up your stamina, I think, are things that everyone should know. Not all have access to such a convenient wealth of knowledge. I think its great for us in general just to know more about this stuff.

3.   Set your own goals: at schools and definitely whilst you are younger, your goals are set for you: "write this essay", "study for this exam", and "go to music class"... etc. I think what the triathlon has shown us is that you can set goals for yourself, ones that seem impossible, and you can achieve them – the will power is amazing. This helps us think about what we want to do with our lives and shows us that we can set our own goals and achieve them.

4.   The importance of family- one of my favourite moments was seeing my mom climbing a major hill in IRONMAN SWITZERLAND on her bike as we all stood there on the top of it! She was all red, with her helmet on, looking so tired but so happy to see us all. It was amazing to see how much of an impact we all had on her being there together and her doing something that she loved.

5.   Always a good story to tell- having a mom who has completed IRONMAN Switzerland AND DATEV CHALLENGE Roth scores as pretty awesome in everyone else's books too! All those lovely things said, it can still be a bit annoying! With 5 kids in the family and Tiffany as a mom I am sure you can imagine we are a competitive family. Having a mom always doing these amazing things can make our little sports feats feel so small! But somehow she manages to make all of us feel great about the sports we play or even the tiny twenty minute runs we do!"

Tatjana:

"7: 30, 23 December, I'm home from university and meet my mom by the door. Together we go outside for a warm-up run followed by some circuits. There is something so bonding about waking up early in the morning and going to workout with my mom. Having been with me since birth, she knows exactly how far to push me, which exercise I will benefit most from and is always giving me helpful advice along the way. I feel so fortunate to have been able to participate in various events with her, whether it is a 6km run or a 3.2km swim. It's incredible to have an experienced ultra triathlete, by my side keeping me calm and always offering words of wisdom (like putting Vaseline under my wetsuit and starting on the outside of the swim to avoid the washing machine). I recently made the mistake of telling my basketball teammates that my mom had completed IRONMAN Switzerland and DATEV CHALLENGE Roth and now whenever I feel like giving up, they remind me that somewhere in my genes is the ability to keep pushing for 15 hours, so I have no excuse. I recently read an article about a man who was a bodybuilder and wanted to experience what his overweight clients were going through in order to truly help him. He completely stopped exercise and began overeating. His wife said that he changed from a person always willing to help to around the house and play with the children to someone who could barely be bothered to move. It made me realise how lucky I am to have a mom who always has energy to be active and do things with us. She applies the lessons learnt during her training to life; I now view studying as a long distance run. Never have I felt that she put her training before me as she always does it in her own time, or includes us in the activities. I think I can speak for all of my siblings by saying that having a role model, who pushes herself like she does, has been such a positive influence on us and has resulted in us pushing ourselves much further than we probably ever would have. She has a unique relationship with all of my siblings and uses sport along the way. This relationship isn't even limited to just our immediate family. She is training for a marathon with my sister and her ex-boyfriend. She came to my university town for a visit with my uncle and ran his half-marathon here. She stuck with him the whole way offering words of encouragement despite the fact that she was running herself. She is an inspiration to all of us."

And Natasja:
How my mom's example as a triathlete has influenced me: "-My mom is always obsessed with listening to your body, which originally, I found very annoying but since my knee operation, she has shown me how to respond to my knee if I have over-stressed it or injured it again and how to start training. If I had listened to her more, I would not have the problems I have. -She has helped me improve my fitness and motivated me to do a half-marathon last April (a small distance in comparison to what she does but I enjoyed training with her and would have not have done it if she was not there). -I eat a lot more healthily because of her recommendations. The meals that she provides for us are good-tasting and full of nutritious items as she uses them for her training as well. -I sometimes do a bit of core strength with her and hope to do more because she believes that core strength is key to my football (soccer) playing. -I understand how to fuel my body a lot more healthily and know a lot of common misconceptions that I hear a lot of friends around me say. -I think it ensured that I respect her a lot more, as she doesn't sit around at home now with all of us out of the house. Her motivation to complete these endeavours is pretty impressive. However, I would not say that it has made me believe that anything is possible (which I think was one of her goals – for us as her kids to believe – when she originally set out on this endeavour). -All in all without her I would be probably six times the size and would pass out after 3km but fortunately she is in my life."

But aside from family there were two other important people without whom I would not have made it, our yoga teacher, Beth and Jaime, friend and masseuse. If the world were populated with more people like Beth we would not be in such a mess. She is American, from Seattle, she is married to Tony, a Spaniard from Valencia. They have two daughters. Among other achievements, Beth is a phenomenal biker, and when they lived in Mexico she used to train with the men's Olympic squad. When they moved to Spain she took up triathlon and was frequently placed in her age group in national competitions. Her husband, meanwhile was a highflying corporate executive. Their life was a normal hectic ex-pat. existence until Tony contracted a tooth infection. Cutting a long story very short, Tony's infected tooth affected his brain stem and within 6 months he became a paraplegic. How Beth, Tony and their family have dealt with this situation has an impact on all those around them. Tony spends four days a week at a centre where he receives much physical assistance and help on a day-to-day basis, ranging from re-learning computer skills to physical therapy. He is picked up by a taxi and taken to Fundación Lescer four days a week. I will never forget when Beth and I dropped in unexpectedly at Lescer whilst on a bike ride. Tony saw

Beth and his eyes sparkled, he reached out his hand slowly to touch her and his face radiated profound joy. He had only left her two hours previously. Their tried and tested love for each other is exquisite. Their dedication to each other and gratefulness for life is a gift for others to behold. As mentioned, Beth is an accomplished triathlete, however an injury meant she had to reduce the amount of activity so she returned to yoga. She had been practicing yoga in Mexico, but now in Madrid, post-injury, she dove into yoga in a way that only anyone who has been intense about a sport can. She followed many courses and became a certified instructor but she was driven by an interest in proving that yoga was also a very important part of enabling endurance athletes to maintain their gruelling training schedules. With her circle of contacts and her determination, she started to write a thesis. This is where our paths crossed. She gave us yoga classes; we in turn became her subjects. She measured us, took photos of us and tailor-made yoga practices for us, taking into account our weak spots, our stiff spots and our training programmes. In short she literally kept us going. We learned so much from yoga; from breathing to opening up spaces and energy we never knew we had. She helped us swim, bike and run better. Her weekly sessions worked wonders for our bodies and mind. Her words of wisdom carried us through the ups and downs both physical and mental. In short, find a Beth!! Be it yoga or regular stretching it should really be part of your schedule somehow, somewhere. It might be that you are very disciplined about stretching, taking care of your own motivation, but if not, recognise that you might need somebody to take care of this side of the build-up. More about Beth later. Finally another important member of the team was Jaime, the masseuse. This is a luxury but a delicious one! Find yourself someone with powerful hands and a lot of experience. It might take a while to find what you are looking for. Once found the masseuse is to be handled with all respect. S/he will understand that taking three weeks off for plantar fasciitis or stiff calf muscles is not an option so will help you work through your injuries. I found myself thinking about my massage on long runs, talking to my legs letting them know that in a few hours, relief would be found on Jaime's table!

GOLD: Welcome this new aspect of your personality. Have to say sometimes I fear being boring, talking about kids, school, family, work, etc., this is at least a new dimension. (I know I can get boring about triathlete/sport/nutrition too!)

SILVER: Try and incorporate your training into your family life. I would often train in a nearby park as Tobias warmed up for and played the first half of his basketball match and then watch the second half.

BRONZE: Think about fund-raising for a charity.

13: Next level of obsessive

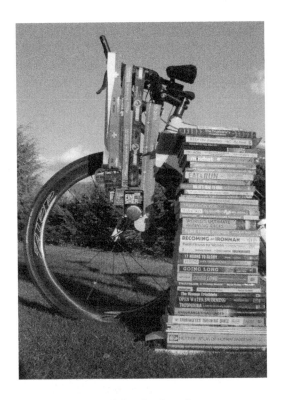

Double the books

"Commitment is pushing yourself when no one else is around."[12]

5 June 2012

24 days after having said to Roland that I did not think my body had an ultra distance triathlon in it, I wrote an email to IRONMAN Switzerland asking when the date would be for IRONMAN Switzerland 2013; the immediate response was July 28th. I was

initially interested in Zürich because I had read somewhere it was a good first timers' ultra tri. I preferred to swim in a lake, the marathon was relatively flat and the biking, whilst hilly, was not terrible. In 2013 it turned out that about 50% of us were full distance virgins. It is hard to describe the emotions swirling around one's head when you are thinking about an ultra distance tri. I can only compare it with being pregnant; thoughts of preparation and training occupied my mind constantly in the same way, as a baby growing inside tends to dominate one's private world. When growing a baby, as the love grows for this tiny person inside, there is always a little smile on your lips because something big and important is happening. In the same way, IRONMAN Switzerland slowly seeped into my bone marrow and I would smile to myself because of the sheer audacity of the challenge.

Summer 2012

With an eye on Zürich 2013, I had two races planned, again the Point to La Pointe, 3.2 km open water swim 2012 in Lake Superior and the New York City Marathon November 4th 2012. Both were preparatory races which, given their time distance away from July, made them C races but given that one was a (horrible) swim and the other a longer distance run, in my mind, I thought of them as B races.

4 August 2012

I swam the Point to La Pointe in 1:21, two minutes faster than the previous year, which disguises the fact that the conditions were substantially less friendly. Something was different; I was in charge this year. My last open water swim had been Buitrago which had had a heroic last 500 metres or so, but this was different. A turning "point" in my swimming had been reached, not that it was not profoundly scary but I managed to avoid the almost overwhelming urge to quit in the first 5 minutes. I was still no mermaid, but I was learning to deal with the fear, and to deal with it quite effectively. Given my long distance tri dreams, this was crucial! As I exited the water I hoped more than anything that the next time I swam this kind of distance in an open water setting it would be in Zürich and I would be preparing to get on my bike for a 180 km. Interestingly in this race of the 434 participants 213 were male and 221 were female, I came in 312th.

Maria had qualified for NYC marathon due to her time in the Madrid marathon 2011 so we decided to go too. The honourable element of the NYC marathon is its capacity to fund-raise. The goal for the 2012 marathon was to raise $1,000,000 for every mile, i.e.$26,000,000. I wanted to be part of that and joined Fred's Team, which is a charity fiercely supporting Memorial Sloan Kettering Cancer Centre, based in New York itself.

Training-wise this meant less of a summer off than usual. By August many people had sponsored me so I knew I could not slack off and let them down. I ran 10 km as fast as I could every other day for the months of July and August and also did 2 solo half marathons around the island. We were on vacation so we biked at least 16 km every day because we had the time to take the bikes to the harbour. This was the most training I have ever managed to do during a summer holiday and it was driven by the debt I owed to my sponsors. Feeling virtuous about discipline is one of the drivers for me. I had set myself the goal of these regular 10 km runs and two half marathons and I had completed them. It is hard to motivate yourself to get up while others are still asleep, put on your trainers and run. But once out, on the road, breathing the early morning air, exchanging glances with the squirrels and fishermen, there are few regrets. Back, after the run, sitting with a hot coffee in my hands, sweaty and exhilarated by the morning's training as others are just emerging from their beds, are special morning moments, hard won moments but moments of deep contentment. Back in Madrid I felt pleased with myself for being so disciplined.

September 2012

My main focus for September and October was the NYC marathon. Maria, Kirsten, Anja and I biked our bike trail a few times to our favourite café in Soto del Real and back, that was a 65km round trip. But, mainly I ran. I ran both outside and inside on the treadmill. I went to some Global Training (high intensity aerobics, leaving you super sweaty and with tired legs) classes at the gym. Maria and I completed the leftover swimming classes we had from the 10 we bought in June and I always practiced yoga on Fridays with Beth.

20 September 2012

"We confirm your entry for the IRONMAN Switzerland on July 28, 2013! Event: 2013 IRONMAN Switzerland (e)
Date: 28/07/2013 07:00 – 23:00
Athlete: Tiffany Jolowicz
Registration-ID: 47960887
Status: Confirmed
Payment: 997.50 ChF Balance Due: 0.00"

It was that easy; a few clicks, a credit card and I was in. If ever there were a time to do this, it was this year. The three of us had the time to train and we now had the equipment. We had momentum from our two half distance tris and we were burning to prove to ourselves and to the world (if anyone really cared!) that we could do the Big Boy. It was crazy, it sent my head reeling, it was way beyond anything I ever, ever hoped to achieve athletically in my life, it was nuts and I was so excited. This was not just a decision I took; I spoke to Roland about whether the dates would work for him and the rest of the family. July is always complicated as there are a lot of people going to many places for internships and summer courses etc. so a lot had to fall into place to make this happen, not to mention the hours of training between now and July 28th 2013. My entire life began to revolve around that, from dawn to dusk it was in my head and sometimes between dusk and dawn I lay awake just mesmerised by the challenge ahead. I, Tiffany, mother of 5, ex-Bond trader, very mediocre Spanish speaker, wife of Roland, was about to embark on a journey of a lifetime. Nothing could wipe the smile off my face, not grumpy supermarket cashiers, not huge piles of laundry, not even traffic jams, and I hate traffic.

2 November 2 2012

The 2012 New York City marathon was scheduled for 4 November 2012. Organisers planned to hold the event despite the effects of Hurricane Sandy the week before. On 2 November 2012, my mother called me to tell me the news of the cancellation. This had not filtered through to our family, as we do not own a television. It seemed like the right decision. We had planned to travel on the Wednesday but decided not to go as friends in NYC told us New York was really a disaster zone. Mayor Bloomberg explained that: "While holding the race would not require diverting resources from the recovery effort, it is clear that it has become the source of controversy and division... We would not want a cloud to hang over the race or its participants, and so we have decided to cancel it."

Some of the marathoners who were already there, ended up helping with the clean-up efforts, due to the "Super Storm Sandy" while others chose to congregate and run an informal "Shadow Marathon" in Central Park. Controversy over the cancellation of the Marathon, the timing of the announcement and the repercussions of the decision, including criticism of New York Road Runners CEO Mary Wittenberg, continued well after the 2012 race was meant to have taken place. As a resolution, all who were registered to run the 2012 race were offered three options: a refund; guaranteed, non-complimentary entry to the ING New York City Marathon in 2013, 2014, or 2015; or guaranteed, non-complimentary entry to the NYC Half 2013. I opted to run the 2014 marathon.

November and December saw us continue with a fairly light but regular training schedule because we knew come January we would have to pick up the pace and intensity.

7 January 2013

29 weeks to go, where to start? I am a visual person so I need to write things down. Tatjana is also a visual person and she bought me The Triathlete's Training Diary, introduction by Joe Friel. I planned to document all my training hours in this diary. Just looking at the inside cover filled me with nervous anticipation and a sick feeling at the pit of my stomach, it is a photo of swimmers, hundreds of them in open water somewhere, about to start an event. On page 24 of his Training Diary, Joe Friel has a weekly training hours table. You can calculate how many hours you should be doing, his recommended training hours against his annual breakdowns. The programmes are made up of three base periods each of 4 weeks, followed by the build periods of three weeks and a rest week in between. This is pretty much the skeleton of all the programmes we found

Our programme ended up being somewhat sporadic, but we did the best we could, given the time available. Obviously it was enough to finish the event but we did not break any records and this loose approach to base, build and rest is the evidence of why we did not!

All in all we trained for nearly 600 hours over 29 weeks, approximately 10% of our waking moments were spent training and this does not include any time spent at the bike shop, dealing with equipment or getting to and from training locations; although I always ran to Pilates and to the pool.

Breaking it down further we dedicated 42% of our time to the bike, 26% to running, 16% to swimming and a further 16% to other that I think is a pretty good division of our training. This breakdown is basically close to the time spent on race day at each discipline, approximately 50% bike, 33% run and 12% swim.

Total breakdown of time dedicated to each sport.

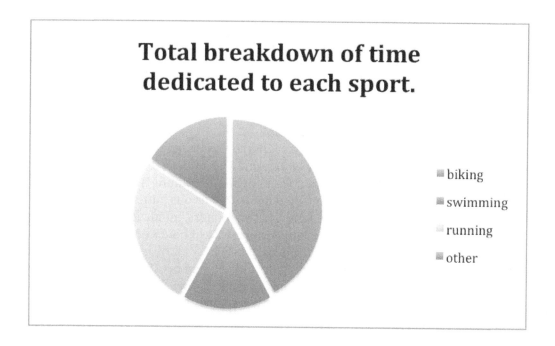

- biking
- swimming
- running
- other

One of the hardest parts of the training is to keep motivated. For some reason the thought of climbing on a bike and cycling 90 km some days just does not appeal or running 20 km or even 5km. Best is to plan in advance so you can prepare yourself mentally, go through the why you should and why you don't want to conversation in your head the day before a long bike or swim or whatever. Training with a bunch of others also means you cannot let them down unless there is an unexpected sick child but for the most part you are very reliant on the other person participating too. There is the other element, never have I ever regretted training! We were always so pleased with ourselves for pushing through. Therein lie mini highs.

As I read through my Triathlete's Training Diary two observations jumped out from many of the pages: 1) hydrate more and 2) stiff legs. I suffered from a tight hamstring for at least a year after Zürich. Now as I look back there is plenty of evidence of it tightening over the training period. The writing was on the wall. Had I read my own journal, I might have learned something! So listening to your body is crucial and definitely a skill to develop. Our ability to listen to our bodies did improve significantly over time. We also learned to listen to each other's bodies so we knew when to tell each other to stop. Training was an emotional roller coaster. As we neared 28 July, we became more and more nervous. Minor setbacks played heavily on us. Not being able to train because of a bad cold one week brought me to tears. On one training ride Kirsten fell badly onto her lower back, the pain was one element to deal with but the fear of not being able to train and losing even a shred of our fitness was heavy. Right towards the end we were doing a turbo training session in my house and Kirsten ran to the bathroom. On her way back, she did not notice that the glass door to outside was shut and so ran right into it. She had passed through that door hundreds of times, she knew full well when it was open and closed. We were not thinking entirely straight. Spot the bump in the photo here, ouch.

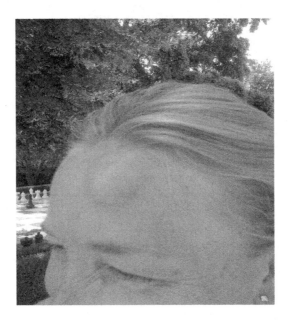

We had set ourselves a C race, Madrid half marathon April 7th, which we completed in 1.59.21, together.

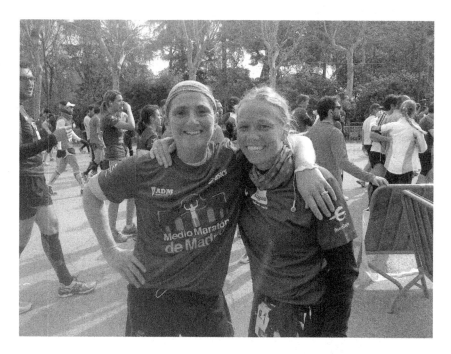

As a B race, three weeks later, we ran the Madrid marathon on April 28th also together in 4:18. We did not intend to run fast because we did not have time for recovery in our schedule but we did want to do the distance. The next day we swam 3.5 km, which felt amazing! That was the first of my 3 marathons in 2013. A good reason for doing these events other than the obvious training benefits is that we learned to cope with the days before. When I ran my first marathon in 2009 I hardly slept the night before. The night before that first marathon I tossed and turned, wresting with the magnitude of the distance I was about to undertake the next day. I kept myself from sleeping, because I was also annoyed at myself for being awake when what I most needed was to sleep. This being my 5th marathon, I had a good night's sleep. With a few more of these events under my belt, the day before, I was learning to eat and drink at times which suited my body and also I began to sleep better before hand which at least made me feel that my preparation was sound.

Over the 10-month training period, we had a couple of epic bike experiences, which shaped our confidence on the bike enormously. For Christmas and my birthday I received two Zipp wheels. According to their web site, Zipp-Speed Weaponry, "Our wheels are the gold standard for performance for good reason. At each rim depth we offer, our wheels provide the greatest aerodynamic advantage on the market." Their wheels are legendary for providing low resistance as they are extensively tested in wind tunnels. In short they make you faster. I needed all the help I could get. Everyone whom I had ever met in the biking world raved about Zipp wheels. They were fixed onto my bike and the brake pads were changed. "Remember," said the bike shop guy, "if you ever put back your original wheels onto your bike to change the brake pads..." Details we were slowly assimilating. We had never experienced a flat tire on a bike outing before. We had seen many cyclists by the roadside dealing with flats and we always asked if everything was ok, not that we would have been much help. But with my new Zipps came a rash of flats: in the space of 4 weeks I had about 12. On one ride I had two so we had to call a taxi to bring us back to our cars. This was frustrating because we would set out to ride long and hard but would have to quit early because of my flat Zipp tires. But most of all it was so embarrassing; my fancy new wheels were a total and expensive disappointment. Embracing the cup is half full mentality, we were becoming very adept at tire changing...down to about 7 minutes and we learned how to use the slick little gas tyre-inflation cartridges. Something had to change. I walked into the bike shop and showed the guys there all my flat tubes. Even with two half distance triathlons behind us, the guys still looked at us as if we were crazy every time we walked in. They joked that we were supposed to ride with our eyes open when on the bike and try and avoid sharp objects. Haha! They checked the current inner tube I had on and said they could find nothing wrong. The break through moment came when I visited my sister Chloë and her husband, Ian. He too had Zipps and he too had suffered. As I was standing in their kitchen a package arrived, he had ordered "anti-puncture tyres." These are of tougher rubber, a tad heavier, not that you would notice the difference but 1000 times more resistant at least. I joke but definitely more resistant. That was the trick; I invested. With my new anti-puncture tyres I have not yet had a puncture in 16 months, but thanks to the weakness of the first tires I sure know how to change a tyre.

In our spare time, we studied the IRONMAN Switzerland website. We poured over the courses, getting to know each one as best one could on a computer screen. I was very nervous about my ability to complete 180 km on the bike. Using an Excel sheet we calculated how many calories we guessed we might need over the whole day and planned exactly what we would eat and where. We got to know the bike route intimately from the diagram. There were 5 relax stations. This is how IM Zürich refers to their water, food, potty stops. Three were named after the villages in which they were located, Grüningen, Forch and Zürich, one was at the top of Heart Break Hill and one had been especially christened the Natascha Badmann Relax Station after the famous Swiss triathlete. Badmann was the first European woman to win the Ironman World championship in Kona in 1998 and went on to win it in 2000, 2001, 2001, 2004 and 2005. On the course we identified two challenges, two steep hills, which we began to fear even on paper. They had been given the intimidating names, the Beast and Heart Break Hill. We visualised the course, especially the Beast and Heart Break hill. Sometimes we allowed ourselves to visualise our finish. It was all just so darn scary.

2 June 2013

Having studied the course of IRONMAN Switzerland for hours; we knew the profiles of the bike and run by heart on paper. We could see the hills and water stations, we knew their names like old friends but now it was time to meet the Beast and check out the Natascha Badmann relax station, to see if Heart Break hill was so bad and look the Zürich Lake in the eye. Kirsten and I disassembled our bikes and packed them into our bike boxes. We boarded a plane from Madrid to Zürich feeling like professional athletes, although I am sure we were not fooling anyone! We stepped out of a Madrid bathed in sunshine and arrived into a torrential rain shower in Zürich. Klaus and Maria flew in from Copenhagen and joined us for this magical weekend. They borrowed bikes from friends in Zürich (they had lived there for 4 years before moving to Madrid.) Also, part of our pack was Thomas and Pepe. Pepe, fluent in 5 languages and a wiry skinny guy is Mr Bike. He is passionate about his biking and fortunately for us a friend of Klaus and Maria's. He takes groups on biking tours around Switzerland and Italy and has recently undertaken an African bike safari to raise money for charity. The rain did not let up so Saturday morning instead of riding the Ironman course, Pepe suggested we take the train South to Lugano. We cycled 90 odd km around Lake Lugano and Lake Como with a stop for a massive bowl of pasta at a wonderful roadside café. The Lugano-Como ride was the most relaxing long bike ride I have ever done in my life. It was not fraught with cadence and carbohydrate worries, we just rode. On Sunday, the rain had just about stopped so we decided to do the 90km loop of the Zürich Ironman. This is the huge spike evident on the Training Diagram on page 49. Thomas who also was a super bike enthusiast joined the 5 of us again. Thomas typically bikes part of the ironman loop in his lunch hour. His familiarity with the route provided us with lots of information. We had an early breakfast and mounted our bikes around 7:30. We rode to the park which we now knew would be the scene of most of the run, (4x10km) and headed off to the Transition area. We began the loop. The first 30km were quite flat but I could not ignore the lake on the left. It was so dark and foreboding and we knew we would have to swim our 3.8km in there in about 7 weeks time. Thus at the Natascha Badmann relax station I was glad to turn left and head up into the hills, away from the menacing lake towards the back country. This ride gave me great confidence. It turned out that the Beast was a 250 metre climb over about 3km, which is not hugely taxing, but enough to piss you off. Heart Break Hill is a steep 100m climb in maybe ½km. The best part about this incline is that it is narrow and on race day, Pepe and Thomas promised me it would be lined with spectators. Having met the Beast and Heart Break hill, having churned up them both, having swung up and down the farmland behind Zürich, I now had a small hope that I could complete this course. Pepe estimated it would take me 7 hours or so…that felt good, but the biggest deal was there was no doubt in his mind that I could complete it. We finished that weekend different people to when we started. There was a change in our minds and bodies. We had biked hard that weekend and we had survived. There was a sensation that we could rely on our minds and bodies in a way we had never been able to before. Our legs were tight and well muscled; they were performing athletically to a higher level now. We were riding distances and speeds we could not even have contemplated a year ago. We arrived pretending to be professional bikers at the airport, now I felt that people looking at us all could see we were preparing for an ironman distance triathlon. I am sure we were still not fooling anyone but I felt enormously invigorated by our success. We returned to our hotel, elated, packed our bags, grabbed a large enough taxi to accommodate our bike boxes and headed for the airport. At the airport we checked in, had a long warm shower and ate a huge salad with yummy carbs. We knew what work was ahead of us but we had a sense that this achievement was almost within our grasp.

In the last 7 weeks, we trained about 100 hours. We were nervous about injuries. My sleep pattern was disrupted with the usual back and forth discussion in my head of whether we had done enough training. I kept thinking, "I will never do this again, it is way too stressful." But on the positive side, I kept thinking, I will probably never be this fit again. I had expected my body to be all muscle, a tight athlete's body; it never really made it to that level. My weight stayed pretty constant over the duration of the 10 months. That was something of a disappointment but we kept telling each other we had exchanged fat for muscle and that must have been the case. Two weeks before the race we had lunch with our professional triathlete friend, Carlos. His closing advice was:

Nutrition; with two weeks to go our meals should contain ¼ carbs, ½ proteins ¼ vegetables, in the final week we should switch to ½ carbs, ½ protein. On a serviette, he drew up a race food plan.

During the last two weeks he advised us to do a 25km run, a 120km bike, a Bric session of biking for 1 ½ hours, followed by a 1 ½ hour run and swim 4km at some point. The idea in the last two weeks or so was to increase intensity and reduce volume. It was to build confidence. Confidence was hard to come by, we were becoming more and more nervous.

GOLD: Work on a mental strategy, by now you should understand your mental strengths and weaknesses. Talk to yourself. Examine your fears now in you mind. Let your mind wander through these fears and dig into them. Better to do this now than on race day. Scan your visualisation library; keep it up to date and ready for the challenge ahead. Remind yourself what gives you positive energy on race day. For me I enjoy interacting with the crowd. People might cheer and shout, "keep going Tiffany," I love that encouragement, I will nearly always respond.

SILVER: Follow your tapering plan to the letter; do not overdo anything. As scary as that feels, it is much more beneficial at this stage to stay lying on the couch, feet up, than to go for a run or bike or swim.

BRONZE: Read chapter 26, to understand that being pretty nervous is very much part of this journey

14: Ironman Switzerland 28th July 2013

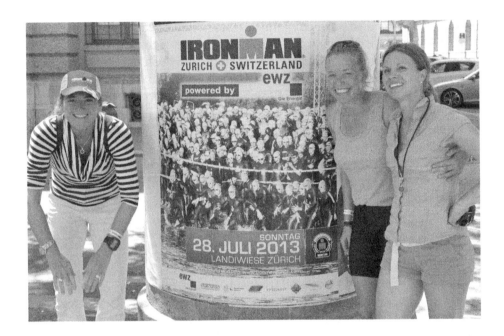

28 July 2013, Zürich

 I rose at 4.30am, exactly as Carlos had told me and ate, the first of the 1000's of calories (a white bread roll with Speculoos and a banana,) I would consume guilt-free all day. Miraculously I crept back into bed and slept another hour. I re-rose and headed for the shower narrowly missing the sturdy wooden bed-leg for about the 15th time since we had been in the hotel. Part of me wished I could just ram my foot against it, break all the 26 bones in my foot and then I could pull out of the race. I was supremely nervous and now I was taking a shower 2 hours before descending into the

Lake Zürich for a one and a half hour swim. I ate another white bread roll with Speculoos (a Belgian/Dutch spread) and a banana. It was not that easy to eat but I knew I had to. All my gear was already at the Transition point so I merely had to pull on my two-piece tri-suit, shoes and a t-shirt. All in all the shower and dressing took about 10 minutes. I went downstairs in search of a cup of coffee and Roland went to fetch the car from the hotel garage. I stood by the entrance to the garage trying to organize my thoughts. Last night we had an early dinner and the whole family wished me luck and gave me a gorgeous golden charm in the shape of the infinity sign. I touched it now, I had a suspicion that the four marathon loops would feel like a never-ending track so it seemed so perfectly appropriate. They had all wished me good luck and gone to bed. As the van appeared from the darkness of the garage I heard laughter, all 5 of them had gotten out of bed to come and wish me good luck, I cried for the first time that day. There were so many emotions whizzing around it was all too much. Trembling with my coffee mug in my hand, we drove to the start area. Triathletes were everywhere. The interesting thing about us triathletes is we come in all sorts of shapes and sizes. Well perhaps I am referring to the Age-Groupers. There is no saying who will finish the day with a medal around his or her neck. Judging our physique will not give any clues but I guess this is a testimony to fitness but also the mind element of this sport. A guy passed me with a t-shirt saying "running is mental." I felt sick!

Time dragged by, we checked our tires, tried to pump Maria's, I think we let out more air than we put in so shaky were our hands and nerves.

The week before we received this email from the event organizers.

"According to the weather forecast we expect temperatures of more than 35 degrees Celsius (95 degrees Fahrenheit) here in Switzerland next weekend. To make sure you are well prepared to race under extreme conditions please note the important information below:

NEOPRENE-SUITS/WETSUITS According to our rules and regulations (www.ironmanzurich. com/athletes/rules-and-regulations) the use of neoprene-suits/wetsuits is permitted up to a water temperature of 24,5 degrees Celsius (76,1 degrees Fahrenheit). We will announce the final decision once transition zone opens on race day. We advise athletes that a non neoprene-suit/wetsuit swim should be expected at all competitions held this weekend.

PREPARE FOR THE HEAT; heat puts additional stress on your body. We ask all athletes to prepare themselves for an extremely hot race day. (Ice will only be provided on Sunday.) Drink enough – during the race but also in the days before. Use sunscreen – apply before the race, after the swim and bike. Wear headgear – fill with ice and put it back on. Use gels and fluids – but little solid food during the race. Take a water bottle at the last bike aid station and cool your head and neck. Use salt – we provide salt sticks on the run course. Cool your body – we offer sponges and ice on the run course. Put sponges under your tri gear to help cool your body. Avoid sun – stay out of the sun in the days before the race.

Please remember: It's about your health and safety on race day. If you have any questions or need more in-formation please contact our staff. If you are feeling unwell during the race, please get to an aid station for evaluation.

All the best for your race! Your IRONMAN Switzerland team."

On reading this email my husband wrote me this, *"Yes you should not mess with this because you have 5 children and me. You will have to be very careful. Sadly the temperature will apparently drop significantly on the Monday"*

At T1, we had no wetsuit to put on as with the high water temperature of 24ºC, it was considered dangerous to swim in wetsuits. After all our training and wetsuit preparation we had to swim our 3.8km without a wetsuit. Of course we had never swum so far in a lake without a wetsuit, so already the day was shaping out differently. Nothing to do now but follow the crowd, focus on the task at hand, because if I dwelled on the unknown I knew I would burst into tears and run away as fast as my legs could carry me.

At 7am precisely the gun went off and the professionals were on their way. At 7:05am, the gun went off again and the Age-groupers, all 900-odd of us plunged into the water. My heart was pumping so fast, my senses were the most alive they had ever been, here I was, Tiffany Jolowicz starting an Ironman. The enormity of the moment caused tears to well up in my eyes again. Big breaths were my only defence against my racing heart. I had done this before in Aarhus, in Buitrago, in Wisconsin. I knew I could beat back my water demons, I knew I was stronger. Time stood still, I glanced around, there were tense expressions on faces, and no one was laughing now. I looked at the lake and it looked back at me with a menacing dark expression. In something of a trance, I let the majority dash for the water and suddenly among them I saw Maria,

111

she was on her way. Seeing her stride so boldly into the water broke my trance, I had to follow her, there really was no other option, so I just walked into the water. I kept left of the masses. I felt no panic and I forced myself to do long, slow, controlled strokes all the time singing to myself. In the week before the race, we were staying in another hotel along Lake Thun and I had had the chance to swim every day in the lake. I think this was the best preparation I could have had, even if I was wearing my wetsuit. In the cold, clear water I had developed a strategy, a simple one, I was going to sing my way around the 3.8 km. The song, which seemed to work for me emotionally and rhythm-wise, was "Jerusalem." Maybe you know it; it is a very British hymn and often sung at school events, in my case always the last day of the school year. So comfortably, on the outside of the group, very inefficiently in terms of distance I began, "And did those feet in ancient times...."

I gained a little confidence and slowly drifted into the main group but quickly felt claustrophobic and decided better to swim further, calmer than get caught in the Washing Machine. Let's face it, I was not going to get to the podium to receive a medal and a bunch of flowers anyway. Continual, unwavering focus on long, clean strokes, long slow breaths and slowly I progressed. I was thinking rowing. Imagining neat oars dipping into glassy water. I again drifted back into the group mainly because I kept having to look up to check where I was going, so I drew some comfort from being in the group because you at least know you are going in the right direction. I got shoved around somewhat but I was beginning to gain in confidence. So much so that I looked for someone to draft behind, why not I thought to myself. I tried and it felt good because I could put my brain on zero, no longer needing to navigate and could concentrate fully on my stroke and my song. As the metres passed, I became a better drafter. My first host drafter suddenly found some energy and moved on, I did not try to pursue because my heart rate was exactly where I wanted it so I looked for another candidate. All this looking around for draft hosts is quite fun and a welcome distraction to the job in hand. I found another candidate and soon noticed that some hosts were better than others to draft behind. It was in the kick some swimmers have high velocity kicks, which create a lot of bubbles; others have tidy, efficient, a pleasure-to-draft-behind kicks. I glided for a while and we came towards shore. We swam under a bridge and I experienced a surreal moment when due to the narrow and shallow nature of the tributary we were swimming through, it seemed as if the entire group was pulling us all along. It was a magical moment when the triathlon momentum generated was significant. We came to the point where we had to exit the water, cross a small island and get back into the water, that was quite hard mainly because I had no idea this was in the course. As I followed the group out of the water I thought I had taken a wrong turn, although I could not exactly work out where or how. I knew I had only swum about 3km and somehow I thought I had missed a buoy and was exiting too early. I looked all around me searching for an explanation; it made no sense to be getting out of the water at this point. I panicked what if I were eliminated in the first hour of my Ironman? I experienced another moment of doubt because suddenly I realised that everyone was descending back into the water. Now I had to get myself back into the water, I had not imagined that I would have to force myself to do two mass swim starts in one day. The momentum of bodies all around me forced me into water. No choice, follow the crowd, not something I typically do, but today I was grateful for the crowd. Back in the water we had about 1km to go. Later I learned that IRONMAN Switzerland is unique because of its "Australian Exit," that is the name given to the manoeuvre we had just been required to make. Had I done my homework I would have found it in various articles. "The swim portion in Lake Zurich features an interesting "Australian exit" between loops over a small island."[13] I maintained for the final 20 minutes and began to think about my bike. I emerged from the water and looked at my watch which said 1.24 which seemed like a disappointing time but as I ran towards my bike, simply because everyone else was running, I figured at least I had survived without letting my heart get the best of me. Experience is definitely the key to survival of the swim phase.

I took stock of my body. My arms felt tired but for the rest at 8.30am in the morning I felt good. I was ready for the rest of my day, my Ironman day. As I pulled on my bike shorts (I always double layer on bike shorts,) I ate one of my rolls. I left the tent and proceeded towards the Bike Park. In my haste, I nearly tripped on a rubber mat, as I approached the Bike Park. Suddenly and abruptly I was stopped at the entrance by a race official. I noticed that he was wearing Birkenstock sandals and had long toe-nails. He raised his hand to bar me from entering the Bike Park. He said, "The rules are that triathletes entering the park need to be wearing a helmet." I saw my helmet dangling on my handlebars about 200 metres from where I was standing. I then realised that it was the only helmet dangling in the Bike Park, also practically the only bike too. "Please," I begged him, I had not come all this way, two and a half years of training to be stopped at T1. Tears welled up in my eyes; my voice began to tremble and my legs began to shake, "Please." I managed to whisper. His face softened, he glanced quickly around him, "Be quick," he said. I collected myself before I crumbled and ran for my helmet, I put it on as fast as I could. I grabbed my bike, turned around and smiled gratefully at the official who waved and gave me a thumbs-up. Hands gripping the handle-bars, I ran next to my bike over the start carpet, heard the click that registered that I started the bike portion, mounted my bike and swung up onto the road.

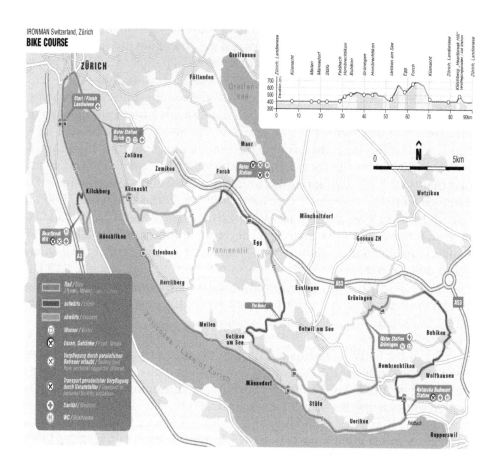

From:
http://eu.ironman.com/triathlon/events/emea/ironman/switzerland/athletes/cours
e.aspx#axzz4YrAz3hqu, used with permission.

As planned, once on the bike I ate two bars and began some serial drinking. The day
was beginning to warm up. The first 20km passed quickly. As I was biking those first
20km I was planning this very paragraph. They were flat, by the lake and I was filled
with the awe of the moment and to be honest I was in awe of myself too. I could see
what we had just swum and my heart was exploding with joy. I was on the second
stage of an Ironman. The first Aid Station, the Natascha Badmann Station came up and
I stopped, dismounted my bike, re-charged my bottles, had a potty-break, smiled

enormously at myself in the plastic mirror and grabbed a banana. I looked forward to being here again in 110 km. Back on the bike, I sipped the Iso-Drink; it was DISGUSTING. Note to all, check what they are "serving" the day of your race, it was just not my cup of tea. I forged on, ate another bar and one gel just before the Beast around km 52. Then around km 59 of the course, you start another windy hill to take you to the highest point at around 700m above sea level. So with two hills and 65km behind me, I pulled into Forch and was met by my sister and brother in law and a very welcome cup of coffee and a second roll. Kirsten's family was also there; it felt so good to see familiar faces. Supporters and family are the best energy boost anyone can have. At this point in the day I had no idea how much I was going to look forward to seeing those beautiful faces as the sun went down. Next followed 60km of pure biking, up and down the Swiss farmlands outside Zürich all the way to Heart Break Hill. I was not disappointed, Pepe and Thomas were right, animated spectators were standing all the way up the hill with cowbells and balloons. I felt like I had won an Olympic medal the way we were cheered and cow-belled noisily up through the narrow corridor. At the top we were greeted by a water station, a hose, bananas and delicious power bars. I tried to drink the Iso-drink but it was not tasting any better.

Up until this point my stomach felt full, almost bloated as if I had over-eaten. I passed one English guy just before the Beast and asked him how he felt, he replied, "Fine except I think I have eaten too many carbs." I had a good energy level because I kept eating every 40 minutes or so. I felt full but was preparing for later on. In my humble, very junior Ironman status, I thought it very important to load up the calories at this stage. Similarly I knew that water was key and worried that with all the stress of the day I might forget to keep drinking.

The best purchase Kirsten and I made was one of our last. It was a Profile Design Aqualite handlebar water bottle with a straw. Nowadays as equipment evolves so fast there are much cooler accessories on the market. What was great about this bottle attached to the handle bars right in front of our noses. Situated right in front of our eyes it was a constant reminder to drink and it did not require groping for bottle. The cool sponge system makes for super easy re-filling and the long straw makes drinking easy although it is a learned skill for sure.

I rode through the start point back by Lake Zürich and started on the second loop, which from Heart Break Hill to the next Aid Station was another 30km. First time I was at Natascha Badmann I thought I would be back here at 110km but I had miscalculated, the second time I pulled into Natascha Badmann I had 128km in the bag as I dismounted the bike to snatch a quick break. This was becoming a routine, fill bottles, grab banana, shower my head with water and potty stop. I knew at the next Aid Station I would see my family. Sure enough at Grüningen there they were.

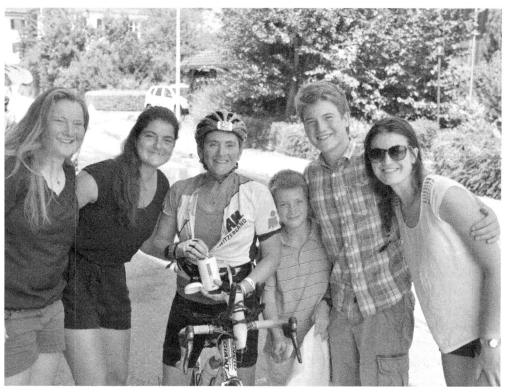
Around 40 bike kms to go

Again such incentive to get to them. We know that long distance triathlon just like other endurance sports is so much about dominating the mental challenge but having family and friends on the course is the ultimate weapon to throw at the mental challenge. Seeing them was invigorating but the best was the two bottles of PowerAde my son handed me. They were an elixir I felt my body absorbing the nutrients and sending them around as for the next 25km I kept sipping from my 50:50 water PowerAde mix. Whatever it takes to keep going, I pedalled on, thinking of all the muscles, organs, fascia, tendons, pumping and throbbing, I felt my pulse and the blood racing around my body as I raced around this course. I imagined my organs and muscles, I pictured them, red and plump and hydrated. Supremely happy, I downed another gel and ground my way up the Beast for the second time. I flew up the second hill just after the Beast overtaking at least 10 people. This was the highlight of the day. I was in, what is known as, the Zone. I felt fit, tight and in good shape. This was very motivating. I felt like all the hill training and turbo sessions we had done were paying off right there and right then. In this state I pulled into Forch for the second time. There was my family again, I am sure it was knowing they were there that propelled me into the Zone. I felt so proud to be participating in an Ironman and so proud that they were there, screaming and shouting, "Go Mama." You could see other spectators smiling at them and me. This gave me so much more energy, I was overwhelmed, I had goose bumps and was shaking all over. I saw Chloë and Ian again, downed half a cup of coffee and my last sandwich, it all tasted delicious. With about 30 km to go I was preparing for a marathon. Up until this point I did not let myself at any point think about the marathon. Every time my mind wandered to the future I pulled it back to the present. No need to worry about the 42.2km yet, it will take care of itself. Surviving the swim had been task one. Only in the last 5 minutes of the swim did I convert to thinking about the bike. On the bike I focused on the stretches between the Aid Stations. I kept reminding myself how incredible this was that I, Tiffany, mother, wife, was actually doing an Ironman. Finishing the bike ride and swim in 10 hours had been the second task. The task of running a marathon in the evening after a 3.8km swim and a 180km bike ride seemed too great to contemplate so I would not contemplate it. However, excitingly, now was the time to start thinking about my legs and the next and final phase. I had taken an Ibuprofen before I mounted the bike and took a second one four hours in as I could feel my left hamstring especially after the climbs. I kept stretching it the best way I could on the bike, meaning on the downhill stretches I always had my left leg long and right leg tucked up. I moved up and down in the saddle in an effort to keep it moving. A Belgian guy passed me at one point saying his back was killing him I handed him an Ibuprofen, he said later that I had, "saved his life!"

At Grüningen, Tatjana had told me that my targeted time for the two disciplines was 9:19. At first I thought she meant 9:19pm, which implied that I would not make the cut-off. I was momentarily confused and scared. Later on the bike I realised I was scheduled to come in well inside the 10-hour cut-off limit with a completion for the two events of 9 hours and 19 minutes. Now I was motivated, I was seriously in with a chance of completing this baby. The bike ride was going well, I felt ok. I knew I could never have achieved this much a year ago. I took off my short-sleeved bike jacket, felt much cooler and raced towards Zürich. With 30 km to go on the bike I tucked into the aero-position trying to keep as low as possible. The last kilometres were long and lonely. Most people were long finished with the bike ride there were maybe 20 of us stragglers. I turned up towards Heart Break Hill and started to pedal up and then out of nowhere sprang Maria's husband and family. Klaus ran up the hill next to me, again tears welled up in my eyes. It is so hard to ride a bike and cry at the same time. Such great motivation; so amazing for being there all day in the heat just cheering the three of us on.

I had not seen Kirsten since 7am that morning and I thought Maria had passed me a while back but I think I overtook her while she was on a potty-break because Klaus and family were waiting for her. I just loved every one of them at that moment. I had 7 km to go. I had never in my life cycled so far and now I had a marathon to run!

As I turned into T2 I heard loud music and a voice booming out of a microphone inviting the winners of the Female Ironman to come to the podium. They were doing the prize giving without me and I still had a lot to do!

During the bike stretch I ate:
3 x sandwiches 2 x Powerbars
2 x Endurance bars 2 x Ovo sports bars
2 x 300-calorie bars Some gum candies 3 x bananas
3 x gels
1 ½ cups of coffee
at least 10 litres of water
2 x Powerades
1 of their disgusting Iso drinks.
Give or take 4000 calories

I parked my bike, there were many more there than when I left 7 ½ hours earlier. I went into the ladies' tent and took off my bike shoes and put on my running shoes and British-flag running vest. I drank some water and ate something although now I don't remember what. A disorientated man came into our tent and started to change. Then he turned around saw all these ladies and ran out laughing. He must have been tired. I found a bathroom and set off again. I gingerly started to run, testing my legs. They worked. At that moment I knew I had another fighting chance. My temperamental left hamstring was ok, my arms moved, my lungs opened up and my quads were lifting and propelling my body forward, I could still run. I ran over a bridge and onto the first of the four 10 km loops. I passed a sign on the pavement, which said 1; 11,21,31, oh man I still had so much to do. At least the temperature was cooling off, during the day it had reached up to 34º I think, which was hot but temperatures we were used to. Training in the hills around Madrid in June/July had at least prepared us for the temperature and taught us to be responsible with hydration. A few training rides followed by headaches, a few training runs followed by salty faces and brittle hamstrings had been

118

harsh but important lessons. I started off half-walking, half-running around the back roads until I came into the heart of the loop which was through the city. We ran past the same lake we had swum in. It all looked very different at this time of day. Lots of tourists enjoying the grassy beaches, families ambling through the streets, trams ferrying people back and forth, restaurants humming and the water tables for the triathletes dotting the loop. In the more populated areas I ran, well jogged. After 6 km or so I saw my gorgeous family again. I slowed to a walk. They were off to find dinner, "see you in four hours," Toby shouted and off they went.

Chloë and Ian situated themselves on the bridge, which meant that for each loop, we saw them twice. They had a huge Union Jack flag and were quite simply fantastic. I don't know how they survived the 5 hours and 23 minutes it took me to complete the marathon. Seeing their faces every 30 minutes or so was the best and also kept me running because there was no way I was going to walk past them. They cheered on not just me but many other happy, tired and almost-IRONMAN Switzerland triathletes. 50% of those participating in this event were virgins, ultra distance virgins! They egged us all on, making friends and giving unrelenting support. There were many other volunteers at the water tables who were just the best. As the day wore on there were fewer people cheering but there were always the happy volunteers handing out bananas, pretzels, warm soup, coke, red Bull and of course water and ice blocks! One British couple who, lived on the third floor of an apartment block watched for hours. The first time I passed, they were sitting in the sun drinking tea and as I passed around 7 pm, they were drinking Gin and Tonics and close to 10 pm, they were sipping coffees. You tend to notice a lot when you are trying to distract your mind from the grind of an ultra distance triathlon marathon! As the kilometres slowly peeled away I began to feel deep elation. I was working my way towards the goal of the last few years. Every once in a while I saw Kirsten whose knee was beginning to play up and Maria who was slowly closing in on Kirsten. She had stomach issues but we were all doing fine. As the evening drew on I could see those who had finished making their way home. They were wearing their glorious finisher t-shirts, which were a great bold blue colour and their medals, chinked proudly around their necks. One finisher shouted across the street to me, "You are going to look so good in the t-shirt!" I saw quite a few with all their gear in the huge black back-pack we had been given the day before, on their back, riding their bikes home. It was now just a question of keeping going. I had 11 km to go, just 11 km was between me and becoming an Ironman, that was enough motivation. After 13 and ½ hours of fight, the head game was over. All I had to do was finish. Every time we passed through the transition area I heard the famous voice of Mike Reilly in the microphone saying " so and so you are an Ironman." I was getting emotional; I was getting so darn close. I passed a guy who was all slumped over; his back was giving him a lot of pain. His wife was trying to help him up some steps; it did not look good. I ran the last 5 km with a German guy who was also doing his first Ironman. His father and sister had run the last 20 km next to him! That was commitment. As I passed Chloë and Ian for the penultimate time, they called Roland.

I completed the last kilometre in 4 minutes and 40 seconds, the fastest kilometre I have ever run in any of my 12 marathons and 30-odd half-marathons. I turned the corner, ran under the big red arch we had passed at 6.50am that morning and entered the final corridor. It was so over-powering that I did not even hear the Mike Reilly announcement, "Tiffany Jolowicz you.are.an.Ironman." I crossed the finish line, my 5 kids running with me. Roland gave me a big kiss and my family, my fellow Zürich-Ironman finishers and friends, Kirsten and Maria and their families surrounded me. It was unbelievable. I was shaking all over. Tears ran down my face. A volunteer fought through the bodies to give me my medal, my IRONMAN Switzerland medal! 15 hours and 2 minutes. Kirsten and Maria looked fresh and happy they had finished 45 minutes before me, running over the line with their kids, holding hands beaming. As Mike, the announcer said, "here come Kirsten and Maria and the whole Kindergarten class."

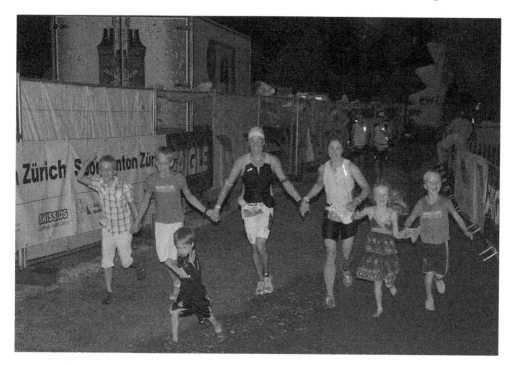

Maria and Kirsten came 1609th and 1610th and I came 1761st out of the 1877 people who finished. It had been a hot day, with temperatures reaching up to 39ºC. More than 300 people who started did not finish, am guessing that the heat beat some of those.

Our respective official times:

	ME	MARIA	KIRSTEN
Swim	1:39	1:52	1:46
Bike	7:41	7:31	7:12
Run	5:23	4:26	4:58
TOTAL	15:02	14:13	14:13

Using the IRONMAN Switzerland official statistics [14] I calculated that: 224 women started the race, 34 dropped out, so drop out rate of @14% 1653 guys started the race, 272 dropped out so drop out rate of @16.5% 1877 people started the race, 306 dropped out, average drop out 16% Draw your own conclusions!!

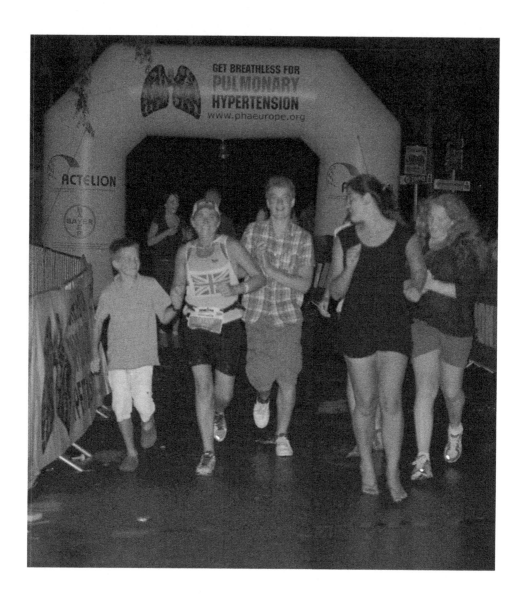

GOLD: Revel, I mean, revel in your achievement; you are AWESOME.

SILVER: Write an account of your day so that when you feel down you can read about how wonderful you were/are.

BRONZE: Take some time off and keep revelling.

CHALLENGE ROTH, JULY 2015

15: Solitary triathlete

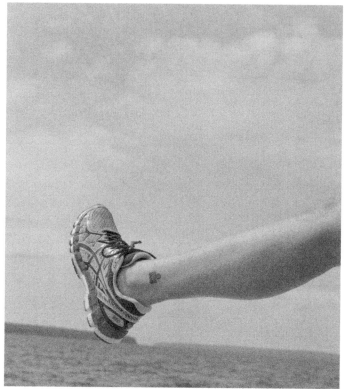

My M-dot tattoo

In the run up to IRONMAN Switzerland, I told everyone who was interested that this would be my only ultra distance tri. The last few weeks had been so unpleasant, the stress had been tremendous, the fears of not finishing and of injury and whether we had trained enough were almost too much to bear. I felt fit but not hollow-cheek fit. I had imagined that my body would have been wirier if it were fit enough to finish IRONMAN Switzerland. I was happy to attempt one, but never in my wildest dreams in early July 2013 did I expect to attempt a second. But then again I had not counted of the mega post-IRONMAN Switzerland high. The aftermath of Zürich was heady. The entire summer I kept replaying the whole day in my mind. On August 10th I watched the Point to La Pointe swimmers come in and burned with pride that I was an Ironwoman, standing there on the banks where I had been a year before, an unsure Ironman wanna-be. The sense of achievement was enormous; I did not have much to compare it with, maybe winning a riding trophy for dressage 30 years previously. When we returned to Madrid in September the earth seemed different as I trod on its surface as an IRONMAN Switzerland finisher. I still had one IRONMAN Switzerland ambition to fulfil. I wanted the M-dot tattoo. I asked a mother at school whom I knew had a tattoo, and she sent me to a parlour in Madrid. Tatjana and I headed downtown and found the shop. We entered and the tattoo artist addressed Tatjana, asking her what kind of tattoo she had in mind. She responded, "oh no actually we are here for my mother!" This time, he grinned and asked me, "What kind of tattoo do you have in mind?" I showed him a picture I had printed from the Internet. "Oh, have you done an IRONMAN?" I grinned back at him, "in that case let's get you that tattoo." It was quite painful but worth every second. It is located on the outside of my left leg, 2 cm above my ankle. Now I belong to another new subset of those on the planet, those with a tattoo.

I still had one event pending in my athletic calendar, the New York City marathon. I had secured my place for 2012 in this marathon by running for Fred's Team, one of the dozens of official charity partners. I had raised money over the summer of 2012 from generous sponsors. The system of fund raising for the official charity partners is excellent. It pits the competitive marathon runners against each other on the charity website and makes them into competitive fundraisers. There is an honour roll constantly posted and it shows immediate updates of donations and who is raising the most. Alongside this, Fred's Team (and I assume) the other charity partners offers prizes over the course of the fundraising period. This generates frenzied emailing to potential donors in order to meet a deadline. The prize I most wanted was a year's supply of Gatorade, but I missed that one. The whole fund raising machine was well managed and well run. Engaged Fred's Team employees armed their runners with materials, stories and tips so that we could contact potential donors effectively. I would have my page to Fred's Team constantly open to keep an eye on the donations rolling in, quite brilliant. I eventually was the second highest fundraiser, which gave me lots of Fred Team stash, much of which I still wear training to this day. It also guaranteed me a spot in the Fred's Team VIP tent on race day. There are over 50,000 participants in the NYC marathon race and we start in waves. This means that we were bussed to Staten Island from Time Square at 6am but my wave did not start to run until 10am. We passed airport type security to enter a huge field filled with tents, Portapotties, coffee and donut stands and VIP tents. It was freezing cold and the queues for the Portapotties were enormous. Everyone was trying to conserve energy but that is hard when you are cold, nervous and thinking, "why the hell am I here." The Fred's Team VIP tent was a godsend because it served coffee, energy bars and best of all, had its own Portapotties. It turned out that my friend Cathy from Calgary had qualified for the NYC marathon because she had run such a fast time in Boston two years previously. We had not seen each other in years as she left Madrid in 2007. The wonderful Fred's Team organisers generously let Cathy into the VIP tent so we passed these three hours hydrating, chatting and peeing, before she ran a much faster marathon than I.

Thus fundraising became a part of my running. I had run IRONMAN Switzerland to raise money for Freedom for Fistula. This is a small charity based in the UK helping African women suffering from Fistula. In their words, "An obstetric fistula occurs during an obstructed labour when emergency care is unavailable. Women suffering from obstructed labour often struggle until the baby dies. During this agonising process loss of circulation causes tissue to die, leaving large gaps between the birth canal and bladder or rectum, causing incontinence. Most women and girls suffering with obstetric fistula are ostracised by their families and communities as they smell and are constantly wet, leaving them to live as outcasts. Fistula is all but eradicated in the developed world. In contrast, it occurs to thousands of women and girls in Africa every day and they have no-one to help." I first heard about this in a magazine article in The WEEK, sometime ago but the story had stuck with me because it was so wrenching. So I set up a Just Giving page and bugged my family and friends again. They generously sponsored me £3,454.98. So in some small way I was giving as well as having a lot of fun. By the time Challenge Roth came around Yoga Beth approached me with a fundraising idea. In 2014 I was not really burning to do a long distance triathlon. Maria moved to Sweden and Kirsten found a full time job, so my playmates were gone. I kept running, I tried to enjoy the lack of structure and pressure, did the Madrid marathon but somehow was not really fulfilled. Slowly I realised what the problem was. 2015 was going to be a busy year, one child graduating from university, one doing her International Baccalaureate and then graduating from High School, Roland was working in Mexico and commuting back and forth from Madrid, I had been asked to give the Commencement address at the High School Graduation and we were moving house from Spain to Switzerland. There really was not much room for an ironman distance triathlon and yet I felt an irresistible pull towards one.

Everyone in the Tri world has heard of Challenge Roth, near Nuremberg, Germany. It is known as Europe's oldest ironman distance triathlon and also the one with the most supporters and dedicated volunteers. To be one of the lucky 5000 to take a place at the start line is legendarily difficult. In 2015, my year, the places available to foreign athletes were sold out in 54 SECONDS and slots for German athletes in 1 minute and 10 seconds. On July 28th 2014, we were in the USA when registration opened at 10 am German time. Despite the odds; I was determined to try my luck at securing a place in the "world's best triathlon." I had set my alarm for 2.50 a.m., but there was no need, I was lying in bed wide-awake with nervous anticipation. So as not to wake Roland, I crept downstairs and opened my computer. The harsh light hurt my eyes briefly. It was so still and dark in the living-room. My heart was in my throat. I logged on the web page and into registration and started refreshing. I imagined the thousands of other people doing exactly the same across the world. The digital clocked turned to 3.00 in the right-hand corner of my screen and I refreshed again. A page emerged and I filled in my personal details as quickly as I dared, simultaneously checking for errors. I sent my data into space. Nothing. It was so weird. I sat and stared at my screen and checked my emails, nothing. I sat there in silence; the anti-climax was huge. I had no idea if I was in or not. I pondered and for some reason checked my junk mail...there it was, I was in. Now my heart really was racing and I laughed at the rudeness of my Hotmail account for putting a Roth Acceptance into junk mail. Trembling I went back upstairs and whispered to Roland, "I am in." I got back into bed and eventually fell asleep with a huge smile on my face, next morning I went for a 5km run.

Nobody else I knew had gained a place at Roth. I was on my own. This meant that I would have to put in most of the hours solo. None of this "ready for the last 5km" or "could never have done it without you." This was really only possible for me because I had already completed Ironman Zürich. I am not sure I could have withstood the crises in confidence totally on my own. In reality, perhaps the hardest part of training for Roth was getting in the hours on the bike. The bike trail, 5km from our house had become an old friend during the training for our first two halves and for Zürich, but motivating my Roth self to ride it on my own was different. Over the 9-month preparation period, I did bike with Beth and Eva (a new Belgian mother at school,) and Minke (a new Dutch mother at school,) this helped enormously but there was no avoiding the century rides that I had to do to pump the miles into my legs. Thus the bike trail took on its own personality. The first 7km are slightly uphill so I knew from the start what kind of a ride I was going to have, based on how my legs and body warmed up. If I effortlessly cruised the first seven, which was unusual, then I would feel stronger in general for the whole ride. I began to gauge my fitness on the first 22 km, which took me up to the highest point of the first part of the ride. This point was called La Cima (translated, "the summit") by everyone who rode this trail and many bikers would bike to the Cima and back for a quick lunch-time work-out. I watched the time it took me over the weeks and months to reach the Cima go down from 1.07 to about 52 minutes. This was quite motivating. I always felt once I had reached the Cima, the rest of the ride was much easier, the fun part, even if I knew I still had 80km or so to ride before I passed the Cima on the way back home.

On the trail I made many new friends, nearly all men who would pass and slow down for a little chat before speeding off again. Many were triathletes, some older men (well into their 70's, they could hardly walk but they could certainly bike,) who went out in groups two or three times a week. I saw these guys often at a café in the Plaza Mayor of El Soto del Real. They would bike a good 30 to 40 km together, have a beer and bike home. I met a guy who asked me if I were Russian, because I was so strong! I met a firefighter who preferred to mountain bike, but was on the trail because he did not have much time between shifts. There was another guy who went out twice a week on his own, (only time away from the Mrs,) who did 100 km twice a week. I saw him often. I pretty much stuck to the same route so that if anything were to happen eventually somebody would find me.

The bike trail became so familiar to me after having pummelled up and down it over three years. The last time I rode it before Roth, knowing that we were moving from Spain as well, I took stock of all it had given me. I had cycled my first distance on this trail, I remember being so proud of covering 44 km the first time we went out. We had laughed and cried on that trail. We had traded opinions on just about everything from world events to child rearing. We spoke of our Tri fears and our love of this challenge. Kirsten had been bitten by a wasp and her face had swollen up. We had changed numerous tires. Whilst out biking, I had learned that my cousin had had a heart attack and died. We had used our tri-bars and my Zipp tires for the first time on the trail. We hated it and loved it. I had learned how to stamp up a hill in the big cog, we had consumed thousands of guiltless calories and braved gusty winds, blistering heat (40ºC) and annoying bugs between the McDonalds starting point and the mountains. We knew the prison on San Pedro, the army base, the beautiful villages of San Agustin del Guadalix, El Molar, Miraflores de la Sierra, Cercedilla and the Castillo de Soto del Real, the old Royal Spanish summer residence. The railway stations and bridges became whey points and gas stations our points of reference and re-fuelling. There was a windy, steep 2km section; I named the "Mont Blanc." Our coffee breaks were always a special part of our trips. The combination of hard work and deep friendship was a great gift. It had been an adventure and the bike trail had been a great teacher. Finally, in preparation for Roth, the bike trail had given me much mental strength and the opportunity to talk to myself. 7 hours on your own, fighting the "why I am doing this demon?" are good ironman distance preparation hours.

I came to regard my rides as either a "do the distance" ride or a "dig deep" ride. The "do the distance" classification allowed me to go out and do between 50 to 80km, usually shorter due to time constraints; they were like maintenance rides to keep the muscle memory. The "dip deeps" were the longer, over 100km rides. I would start to dread these a few days prior. These required mental and nutritional preparation. I had many hours to concentrate, many ups and downs to conquer. I developed different strategies to entertain myself. One included rehearsing an important speech, the Commencement speech at Natasja's High School Graduation. I wrote and re-wrote this speech on these rides. I also gave it out loud to the roads, the trees, the up-hills and the tireless white line. These rides took a lot of energy, they made me dig deep, but they were of course the most rewarding.

Given that I was training alone for Roth, I thought it would be a good idea to do Buitrago half ironman distance for a second time as it was so close to home. I assumed that as I was well into my training for a full distance I would have an easy and enjoyable time over the half distance that I knew so well. I was not looking forward to the swim, as it had been a while since I had swum in open water but again it was only 1.9km so surely I could dominate the distance. Somehow over the past few months, I had managed to burden myself with plantar fasciitis in my right foot. It was annoyingly painful when I ran over 10 km, fine when I biked and swam. So the half marathon at the end of the Buitrago half was going to have to run itself based on a song and a prayer and my new insoles. I fervently hoped that Buitrago would give me confidence on the bike as I had done considerably more biking than ever before to keep my fitness from slipping without the running component.

GOLD: Definitely get the tattoo. If I were to do it again, I would place it on my left calf half way up my leg so it would be seen by runners behind me. No one sees it at the side.

SILVER: Give your bike ride trail a personality. Name various spots or stretches. Love them and hate them.

BRONZE: Take one section of this ride and time how long it takes to do this stretch. Keep a record and see your times improve. You can also do this for a running stretch you often cover and of course you can do it in the pool. Every so often time yourself over say 100 metres.

16: Winning my age-group at the Buitrago Half

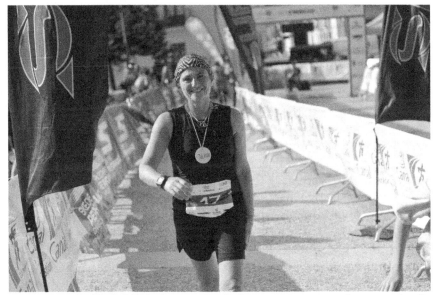

La "meta" (finish) Buitrago half, it was not exactly crowded!

14 June 2015

13 pink caps (the female participants,) lined up behind professional athletes and paraded down to the water's edge. There is a lot to be said for smaller scale events, the logistics are much simpler. I was right at the back, as the oldest. The swim directions were complicated, as we had to be on the right side of one buoy and the left side of another. Spanish instructions tend to make everyone confused and here was no exception. I thought I understood but was not overly worried if I had not because I did not expect to lead the pack.

Waiting to start the swim always saps me of energy. Standing at the water's edge with the day ahead of me I just wanted to disappear. As had been the case in 2012, Buitrago started at noon so I had had the whole morning to toss the stupidity of the day around my head. But today was different because there were many familiar faces on the course. Not only was Sacha's (now ex-) boyfriend, also doing his first half ironman distance but we had two relay teams taking part as well. Tatjana (daughter) swimming, Ian (brother-in-law) biking, Maria (Ironman friend) running were the "just tri-ing" team and Tom (Sacha's friends, Karolien's (now ex-) boyfriend) swimming, another Tom (husband of Eva, my biking friend,) biking and Kirsten (Ironman friend) running were the "just 4 fun" team. A little confusing I realise but the point is that we were a whole group of friends taking part and a bigger group of cheerleaders supporting.

Off we went, my heart rate rocketed and I started singing my song in my head. This should only take 45 minutes I reminded myself and then I could get out on the bike terrain I knew so well. It was a very slow 45 minutes. As the pink caps passed the penultimate buoy on the left, the first men started catching us up. The men had started 8 minutes after us. Everyone was respectful; there was minimum pushing and shoving even as we exited the water onto a very unstable floating white platform. I ran up the steep hill, which was covered with sand to protect our feet. I was somewhat nervous for my foot because it was still fragile from the plantar fasciitis injury I had been desperately trying to get to heal. This woody, steep, stony terrain was exactly the type that would tear the muscles of my slowly healing foot.

I started pulling off my wetsuit as I ran up the hill. There really was no reason for me to be hurriedly pulling of my wetsuit, it just seems to be standard cool during a triathlon. In T1, there were only 4 women's bikes left in the rack so I spotted mine without a problem. I fought to get the rest of my suit off and rustled through my gear to fish out my biking shorts, gloves and top. I grabbed my bike, checked my water bottles and headed out. I left T1 and passed over the timing carpet to the cheers of my family. Their loudness caused others to join in and shout. Distracted by their noise I was not paying attention to the 10% incline, which was the start of the bike ride. This was tough to ride up from zero and later my sister, Chloë told me that many bikers had toppled over right at the start. This hill took a good 3 minutes to conquer, then short and flat and then 2.5km up to the 35km loop I knew so well. Somehow all this climbing, which really was not that steep, kept my heart from settling and I felt tired from the start. I told my legs that usually felt warmed up around the 50km mark to keep doing their job and to hang in there. Not sure they were convinced. This is the mental part of the race. I was trying to change the way my body was feeling but frustratingly, my body was winning. My legs pushed and shoved me around the course, we completed the first loop but it was just a drag. In the second loop I took my time, I was not going to break any records today, so I just tried to conserve the strength I had in my legs as it was obvious that the energy I had had on my practice rides was not going to be released on the bike today. I could only think that my legs had not really recovered from two turbo sessions at the weekend and the hard ride the Tuesday before.

I arrived in T2, 3 hours and 15 minutes later, just 15 minutes faster than 3 years previously. I was disappointed, but with a half marathon ahead of me, now was not the time to dissect my bike ride. I reminded myself that it was just a training day. Having not run more than 10 km in the last 6 weeks I was a little nervous about my performance but just had to rely on the running I had done in the last 20 years to propel me around the course. The run was more trail than anything else. I felt like I still had a lot of work ahead of me, but I had been fighting myself all day so I figured I could keep this up for another 2.5 hours. I made myself a deal, walk up the hills and the treacherous, stony downs, and run the rest. Slowly the kilometres began to add up, 1, 3, 5 and then 6. I got to know the terrain and route a little. I finished my first loop of 6 km as most were finishing their second loop. Just 9km to go. I imagined the photo that could have been taken of me as I ran off into the sunset pretty much on my own except for a handful of guys behind me.

Roland, my brother, Kingsley and his wife, Audrey and Aleks had positioned themselves at a strategic water station, so Kirsten, Maria, Jaap and I passed them about eight times during the run. Aleks shouted and screamed as I ran past and ran some of the way with me. With 7 km to go they left for the finish line and I began to feel the warm happiness spread through me, the warm happiness that goes with this crazy activity and keeps you coming back for more. My butt was hurting. It is usually my legs and/or quadriceps, which start to complain first, but for some reason on this Saturday afternoon, it was my butt. However looking for the silver lining, which is paramount in this sport, I was supremely glad that it was not my right foot.

On the bike I had seen Tom and Ian and on the run I had seen Kirsten and Maria, it was just like old times, their beaming but concentrated red sweaty faces a loop ahead of mine! These events are gruelling but the moments on the race when you pass a fellow triathlete and you recognize their pain and just underneath the grimace you see their solid determination, you can not help but exchange a salute of respect, a knowing nod of empathy as we all chase this strange dream.

133

I ran 3 km further and almost bumped into a race organizer with a walkie-talkie. "Te estamos esperando," " we are waiting for you." The Buitrago tradition is to present the medals at 7:15 once all the participants are in. "Voy corriendo," I responded, "I am going as fast as I can!" I ran past the medieval wall next to a happy, bouncing Aleks and into the finishing chute. My crowd of 15 fans started cheering, shouting, screaming somewhat disproportionately loudly compared to the speed of my accomplishment, but all the noise generated more shouting from all those milling around the finish line. I won my category; I was the fastest female 50-55-entrant....and the only one! In Spain they categorise age groups according to the year of your birth, not the actual birthdate so although I was not technically 50, I was competing in that age group. It is always a wonderful feeling to run into the finishing zone; it never lets you down and that finish was no exception. It had been a long hard fight around Buitrago. I had expected it to be easier, I knew the territory, I was supposed to be almost fit enough to do an ironman distance triathlon (in less than a month,) and there were lots of people cheering for me. But I finished, my mind won over my weary body and the finisher's glow was warm and enveloping. Still, the night was but young. We had 27 people for dinner, Sacha's ex-boyfriend, and his parents, the team members of "Just tri-ing" and "Just 4 fun," their families and of course my family. We had a lot of celebrating to do, namely finishing a first half ironman distance triathlon and "Just tri-ing" came in third in the relay competition. We collected my bike, went home, showered, charged our glasses and dug into well-deserved paella. It had been a wonderful day.

GOLD: Look at the course map and select the best vantage point for your spectators in advance, estimate where and when you will be at certain spots, mark them on the course map, that way they will enjoy the day and want to come to support you again.

SILVER: Take good care of your supporters; make sure they have water and snacks and a camera. Often races have a tracking App, download this for them, enter your race number and get them prepared.

BRONZE: Take a B event like Buitrago and make a social event out of it. The Buitrago half was an excellent training event but was also so much fun.

17: Countdown to Challenge Roth- my second ultra distance tri.

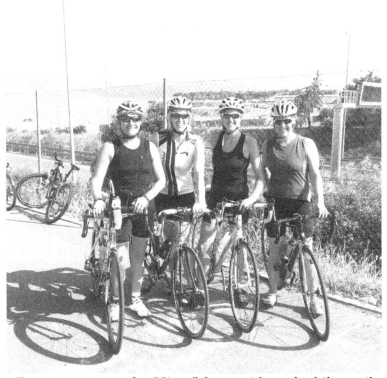

Fun moments at the "Cima" (summit) on the bike trail
with Minke, Eva and Beth

Training for Roth, I basically followed Christina Gandolfo's Ironman Training Program from her book, The Woman Triathlete, with some of my own tweaks. For the running, I ran 3 half marathons before Roth. The furthest distance I ever ran in the 10-month preparation period was 28km. I did more turbo running than I had ever done before. Turbo running for me would be going out for an 8km run. I would try and complete a kilometre at an average pace of 5:15 km/hr. This is pretty fast for me, like breathless fast. Then I would walk, take a break for 30 seconds to 2 minutes depending on how breathless I was and then run the next kilometre at the 5:15 pace. Sometimes I would manage 10 km like this. On the days I could not face running, I would speed walk 12 or more km over as many hills as I could find. Other days I would run to the biggest hill in our area which was 600 metres long and maybe a 6% incline and run that 10 times. I also ran a lot of fast 10 km, fast for me being 52 to 53 minutes. This way I would vary the task at hand a little. For about 10 Sundays Natasja and I did some longer runs of around 15km.

For the biking alongside the longer bike rides, which I gradually increased up to 142km, I became the queen of turbo. Building up from 35 minutes to 1.05 hours I would work very hard doing this at least twice a week. Mostly I would follow this with an easy 5km run. These turbo bike sessions were big sweat, big heart rate workouts. I could feel my gums pulsating and my heart rate would be up around 185 beats per minute. I spent more time on the bike because of my plantar fasciitis injury. I was fastidious about icing it especially if I went for a short run after biking. Experience has taught me patience and respect for injuries. These harder turbo workouts whilst tough, sometimes they made me feel like throwing up, were interesting because as my fitness increased, I felt able to push myself harder, to the next level. Just as with the turbo running ladder, a bike ladder has a similar build-up and down. In the beginning I would pedal hard for 15 seconds with 15 seconds rest, then pedal hard for 30 seconds, with 15 seconds rest then 45 seconds hard pedalling, 15 seconds rest, then 30, hard, 15, rest, 15 hard, 15 rest. As I became fitter it went to 30, 45, 60, 45, 30 with 15 seconds rest in between to 100, 120, 150 seconds and back down. Obviously I was becoming fitter but also I got used to dealing with the pain, the pushing and the pulsating heart rate. As much as I hated these ladders, I loved them too.

On the swimming, I swam at least once a week and at least 1.75km each time. I swam when Aleks was at swimming training, so had 40 minutes from start to finish, thus, I did not have time to dawdle! When I had more time I would do a 3 to 4km swim. I never really pushed myself hard in the pool; it was about doing the distance and focusing on deep, long, efficient strokes.

The suggestion for fundraising came from Beth our yoga teacher. She suggested running Challenge Roth to raise money for Fundación Lescer, the facility that cares so well for her husband, Tony. Fundación Lescer is not a slick fundraising machine like Fred's Team or JustGiving. Fundación Lescer was always in need of money, (especially after the Spanish government cut funding for private rehabilitation centres) staffed by medical personnel not young techies writing programmes and processing credit card donations. I set about training, Beth set about helping the overworked administrative staff understand the world of fundraising. It took about 7 months but they did it. There were a few hiccups when we went up live for donations, but in the end, we managed to raise €26,000 for Fundación Lescer. Tony and Beth are the kind of people that make that kind of venture happen.

Training for Roth was tricky for three reasons: 1) because I was training on my own, 2) we were moving country and 3) I had no idea of the terrain except from the Challenge Roth profiles I found on their web site. The only one of these three I could change was number three; knowing the terrain. A week before the actual event, Aleks and I drove the 475 km from Luzern to Roth. There we met Roland, who had flown in from Mexico and Tatjana who had flown in from somewhere but I do not recall where. On Saturday 4 July 2015, the hottest day ever recorded in German history, I biked the 90km loop of the Challenge Roth bike course, on my own. Afterwards, I went for a brief but welcome dip in the Danube Canal, the venue for the swim. I wanted to meet the water and talk to it. I did not put my head in it and swim that was a mistake. I saw the fields where the event was to be held and where T1 would be located and the park, which would become T2. Roland picked my bike and me up; we went out for dinner and drove home the next day. I now knew what Roth looked like. With a week to go I focused on the mental preparation as time had run out for any physical improvement.

In our new house in Switzerland we hoped that the summer heat would abate somewhat. That was not the case, Switzerland too was experiencing an energy draining heat wave. Coupled with the weather, my age was catching up on me. I was to turn 50 on August 1 2015 and July 2015, menopause started with relentless, debilitating and embarrassing hot flashes. The only respite came when Aleks and I went down to Lake Luzern at around 5pm most evenings for a delicious swim. I fought into my wetsuit and let the cold water give some relief. Aleks in his canoe with me swimming beside him was very calming and the water was very cooling. He coached me, kept me working hard to the last moment, "just because you only have 300 metres to go, does not mean you can slack off." I put the heat and hot flashes out of my mind and concentrated on slow, long, rhythmic strokes, like oars from the rowing boats we could see around us. Striving to emulate the unhurried, technically perfect strokes; I gave myself up to the swim. Using visualisation to overcome ragged emotions. The last swim before going to Roth, Tatjana swam with. It was a glorious evening, the "Golden Hour" in photographic speak and a swim I really enjoyed. It was a good last swim.

As I continued with the moving paperwork, e.g. residency registration, new school documents, driving licenses etc. my hot flushes got worse. What, why now? I was miserable in those last two weeks. It was so hot I felt like I was never hydrated. One day the temperature went down to 27°C and Aleks and I went on a short bike ride. Well there was some energy in my legs, which gave me a little hope. Always swirling in my triathlete mind was "have I done enough training?" My body felt strong sometimes and just plain flabby at others. Sometimes I felt I was winning the fight against the slow ageing process and other times I knew gravity was dragging me slowly as my body became slacker and slacker. The stress of the last few weeks was weighing on me. Some people never move house, let alone country; some people never do a marathon, let alone an ironman distance triathlon. Some people might tackle an ironman distance triathlon but not at 50 and not in menopause, who did I think I was? The move was so fresh, I felt like my body was in Switzerland but my head was still in Spain. I had to get my body and head to be together. That is what I did in the last few days. I had no choice. Thank goodness I already had one ironman distance triathlon in the bag so I knew more or less what lay in store for me. I rested, moved slowly, talked to myself, visualised the Danube Canal and the swim, the villages I would be passing through on the bike course and the run course I had seen on-line. I dared to let the thrill of the finish dangle in my mind. Thankfully, somehow it all came together. Maybe doing an ironman distance triathlon at this age had given me some wisdom and a different kind of self-confidence and self-understanding. By the time we left the house on that Thursday morning, I was ready; well I had to be right? Only I could prepare myself properly, only I could drag myself together. I had packed over a period of about a week, making piles of gear, checking the piles off against a printed out list a neurotic six or seven times, making sure that I had everything. Thursday morning, early, Aleks and I drove back to Nurnberg, a lamb to the slaughter.

The next morning, Friday, with 48 hours to go, Aleks and I went to the Tri Tent in Roth to pick up my registration pack. This was Chrissie Wellington country; she was everywhere. She had broken the world record for the fastest female three times in a row at Roth. It currently stands at 8.18.13. The fastest time ever recorded for an ironman distance triathlon also is held in Roth, in 7:41:33, Andreas Raelert won his debut Roth in 2011. For me these times are mind-boggling but the privilege of competing on the same course as these greats is an inexplicable experience. Chrissie was in my mind all Sunday as I ploughed through the same water, cruised over the same roads and pushed my body through the streets of Southern Germany.

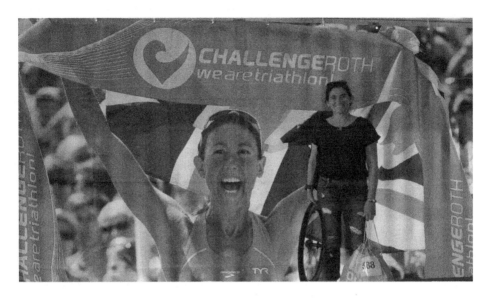

My hero, Chrissie Wellington

We picked up my number, bags and goodies and sauntered through the Expo and breathed Tri air. We bought a pair of running shoes for Aleks and two new tires for me. I was aware that even though I could spend the entire day at the Expo, the 12 year old who was so willingly trotting beside me needed some other entertainment. We left Tri Country and drove to the Playmobil Fun Park, which is close to Nurnberg. We headed straight for the cafeteria where I ate a giant plate of plain pasta. Then we roamed through the Quarry, the Pirate Ship, the Knights' Castle, the Octa Climbing, the Wild West and Noah's Ark. After hours with Playmobil, we went to find Chloë and Ian at the Hipoltstein campsite. The campsite is located by the Danube Canal, across from the swim start. The field I had seen the weekend before, had become a beehive of activity. Many athletes stay here for the weekend. Chloë and Ian checked over my bike, tightened screws and changed the tires for me. What a luxury to have a technical team at my disposal. We ate a delicious carb meal and then Aleks and I headed back to our hotel. Roland, Tatjana, Natasja and Tobias arrived late that evening. The following day, Roland, Chloë, Ian, the kids and I toured Nurnberg, specifically the Nurnberg Trials museum. I ate another plate of pasta and dropped my bike off at the bike park and cast an anxious glance at the Danube Canal and all the preparations being put into place. There are over 6,000 generous and very well organised volunteers contributing to the slick running of Challenge Roth. Kirsten had promised to come and support and she arrived just in time for dinner. I went to bed early. All day and all night, I drank as much Gatorade/water mix as I could handle.

GOLD: Be prepared for the mental battle. It is fierce and draining, even if you are not menopausal, not moving house or close to the venue.

SILVER: On the other hand you have to enjoy the run up to an event such as this. You are fit, probably more or less injury-free, about to embark on a day in your life that you will remember forever. So embrace all the sensations, record them if you are a diarist, or take photos.

BRONZE: Use a checklist as you pack each bag and load stuff into the car.

18: 50-year old takes on Europe's oldest long distance triathlon, Challenge Roth.

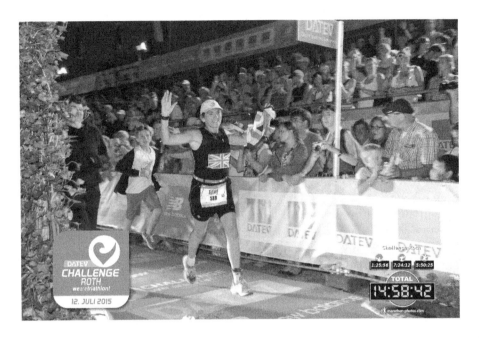

Finishing Roth: Photo used courtesy of marathon-photos.com

12 July 2015. I was in the 6.55 wave. I felt sick to my stomach. I had not slept well; I had had food at 4.30 and some coffee and a bagel and Speculoos in the car on the way in. 5,300 athletes participated in Roth 2015. There were 3,400 single starters and 660 relay participants. Why was I here again, why was I putting myself through this? I made my way to the water's edge with the other 200 women in my wave. Once in the water I stuck to the right of the canal. There was not much room so I let the others move in front of me and I tried to keep my heart rate down. I knelt down and put my head in the water. It was incredibly cloudy; I could see nothing ahead of me, not even a

pair of feet to draft behind. It was like swimming in fog. Allowing only positive thoughts to enter my head, I reminded myself that the best thing about the swim at Roth is that it is up a canal on the right hand side, all the way to a bridge, around buoys at the end and back down the other side of the canal, it is basically straight so no worrying about drifting off into the middle of nowhere because you just bump into the side of the canal, like a bowling ball hitting the side. It is a question of putting your head in the water and swimming straight for an hour or so. I started to swim, it took me ten minutes or so to get used to the lack of visibility. That is the nature of triathlon; you just never know what it will throw at you. When I had been in the canal the week before after my 90km bike loop I had not put my head in the water, never imagining that it could be so difficult to see. I settled into my routine, my song in my head, my long gentle strokes, my controlled heart rate and I just swam and swam and swam. I will not say it was pleasant but I felt in control of this swim. Just as I was approaching the finish some of the faster men started to catch me up, but all were polite and I emerged in good shape. I dashed off to find my bike. The atmosphere at Roth is fantastic. The streets around the Danube Canal were lined with thousands of supporters even at this early hour on a Sunday morning. They are known for the Roth wave, which is a sign of respect for the athletes. The wave is performed by the supporters. In 2015, there were over a quarter of a million of them lining the entire course. For the wave, they stand in a line and do a kind of Mexican wave as the athletes pass by and accompany it with a long wooo sound. It cannot but make you feel special and a little in awe of yourself!

I had survived the swim, which is such an overwhelming feeling because the swim remains so scary; I still did not feel I could completely rely on my panic suppression. I channelled my excitement and positive vibes into biking leg energy. The whole day ahead, my second ironman distance triathlon, I was soaring because it was here and now and mine to grab. I crossed the bridge and saw Chloë and Ian and Kirsten. I, Tiffany Jolowicz was a real live triathlete. I was still far enough ahead in the pack to look like a relatively fast triathlete too! The public adored me.

Over the bridge and around the corner, up the incline, the crowd thinned out and the hard work started. I began eating. The strategy of Zürich was to be the strategy of Roth. Passing the kilometre signs can be quite disheartening in the beginning. At around 5km I passed the 90km sign, which made me grimace. At around 65km I passed the 150km, which seemed to be taunting me. You pass the longer distance signs because, as is the case in Roth, if you are doing two loops of the same course, whether it is biking or running, the signs for the second loop are already in place. I had a whole 85km before I would be back here and then I would still have 30km to go. The distances seemed impossible again. These are the dig deep moments for which you train. Fortunately, the aura of the day is enormously motivating and Roth has a special atmosphere. At 82km I passed the 170km sign I waved at it, assuring it I would be back soon. I buckled down, pedalled, ate and drank. Four hours later, I sailed past an enormous grin on my face. Now between my medal and me stood 20km on the bike and a marathon. Piece of cake. The bike ride was long but had great moments. I will never forget forging my way up Solar hill, its thousands of spectators lining either side leaving just enough space for the bikers to ride up in single file. It was a Tour de France moment and one of the highlights of ironman distance triathlon worldwide. As I pumped my way up the second time, my legs tired but still working I emerged at the top with tears streaming down my face. The emotion of ironman will always be heady. I did feel like an old lady on my bike as the stronger cyclists who had been trapped behind me up the narrow hill fanned out and sped off into the distance. I passed Chloë and Ian for the second time on the bike, had another cup of coffee with them and continued. I saw Roland, the kids and Kirsten twice on the ride and a gentleman dressed as a clown, with bright red lips, about 6 times. After a while I thought I was hallucinating he turned up so often.

Seven hours and 24 minutes later, I biked into T2 and was met by throngs of volunteers who were helping athletes strip, change into their running gear and apply sun tan lotion. My helper, with her thin, efficient hands, unpacked and packed my bags, tied my shoelaces and with her reminder to go to the bathroom on the way out made me laugh out loud. Service was first class; they were like nannies chasing the children to play outside. Before I even knew what happened I was starting the run. I ran down into the wood, which led to the Danube Canal loops. As I was beginning my run the stronger age-groupers were finishing their Challenge Roth 2015. They all looked deadly serious and were concentrating hard. Once on the running trail, the water stations were plentiful, and the volunteers brave because the fruits they were offering were attracting lots of wasps. My loyal family had settled themselves around km 8 so I saw them twice on the first loop and then again around km 24, so I saw them twice on the second loop. Every time I ran passed them it was so uplifting, they cheered and shouted, "Mama," it was so emotional, I love crying and running; I felt so special. It began to get dark and I was tiring, walking quite a lot. I went to the Portapotty about 8 times on that run. I ran for a while with a woman from Frankfurt and then another guy from the Ukraine. Faces became familiar, running styles too. There is camaraderie on the last stage of an ironman distance triathlon second to none. Everyone is grinding away at the distance and faces slowly become more and more animated. The pain of tired legs is right below the surface but the moment of extreme happiness is closing in rapidly. Thirteen hours after the starter gun had gone off, there were not so many of us left out on the trail as we doggedly half ran half walked. This is known as the triathlon shuffle. I walked up an incline and over a bridge and heard, "There she is," and then "Come on Tiffany." It was Chloë and Ian and about two other supporters still out there. I dragged myself to a run and responded, "I am flagging." They responded, "see you at the finish." Magic words, I kept repeating them to myself, "See you at the finish." With 2 km to go I was in the town of Roth. Once again and for the last time on the course I saw my awesome family. They were still shouting and cheering, "Come on Mama." They had been supporting me since 10am. Onlookers smiled at me and at them, I was bursting with pride. They had been out and cheering all day long. What had I done to deserve such a great group of people around me? It had been a hot day and they had never considered taking a break.   On the bike and again on the run, they had staked out a great spot where I could see them on numerous occasions. I loved them all so much at that moment. I forged on; I could hear the madness at the stadium. I slowed to an even slower walk trying to commit everything to memory. I was fairly certain I would not do another full ironman distance triathlon again, so I wanted to remember this feeling forever, to capture my achievement in my body so that I could always call on this strength when I might need it. The moment I had been training for was about to happen and I was ready to be transported into the hot, throbbing atmosphere of the Roth Stadium. Up and down, around and through and then suddenly I was there. Chloë handed me a Union Jack and I carried it into the roaring arena. Behind me running were the kids and Kirsten. It was crazy, crazy and delicious. The energy surged through me as I ran under the timing arch, 14.58. Two years older and four minutes faster, thanks to the T2 helper I am sure. A volunteer came up to me congratulated me and ceremoniously hung my medal around my neck. It was gold with black, yellow and orange, with a retro feel about it. It was heavy, just as it should be. The moment was enormous. Roland and the kids, Chloë and Ian and Kirsten were all there. Another finisher kiss from Roland, I was so thankful to all of them for supporting me all day. I went to the finishers' tent and had the biggest cheese roll I could find. I love cheese rolls and this was one of the best I have ever had, perfect combination of crunchy and soft bread, no skimping on the cheese. Fellow finishers congratulated each other, embracing new-found friends fresh from the trail. The atmosphere of achievement was heavy in the air. I followed my new friends to the t-shirt pick-up. I could feel my legs stiffening. The pain was not however going to wipe away the smile on my face. I picked up my t-shirt and headed off to find my bike. The hour after an ironman distance triathlon is a glorious hour. The concentration of the day, the stress of the training and the feeling of pride all mesh into one surge of perfect self satisfaction. There are plenty of moments of self-doubt in life, low moments for one reason or another, but the post ironman distance triathlon high has taken me twice to a place of extreme happiness. I recommend it!

	Roth 2015	Zürich 2013
Swim	1:25	1:39
Bike	7:24	7:41
Run	5:50	5:23
Total	14.58.42	15:02.43

Comparing Zürich and Roth, looking at the differences in the swim, bike and run times for each ironman distance triathlon, you see how the training had an impact. The improvement of 14 minutes in the swim shows the gain in confidence in two years. The biking gain of 17 minutes is as a result of more focussed training, i.e. the turbo sessions and the run clearly shows that I neglected this in training, mainly due to an injury and lack of time, I figured I would be able to push through on the marathon stretch if I managed to get that far and that is what I managed to do, just push through.

GOLD: Plan your finisher photo; (remember the photo of Jane Tomlinson on page 23) leave about 2 seconds between you and the person ahead of you in order to get a clear finisher photo with just you on it. In Zürich, the guy right in front of me hogged the photo, by Roth, I had learned my lesson, the camera caught just me on the image. You don't want to share that frame with anyone else.

SILVER: If you are of the belief that hairy armpits ruin a finisher photo, then shave your armpits a few days before the race.

BRONZE: It is much, much easier to go to a triathlon event by car than by plane

19: Skiing accident

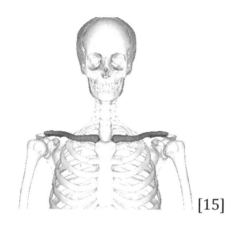

[15]

Am not exactly sure how it happened, well actually I am. At 50, you would have thought that I would be through the days of reckless, I-can-do-it-in-any-weather skiing. Surely that is a teen behaviour. It was the last day before Natasja went back to work so we decided no matter what we should ski. We drove the 25km to our local mountain. The weather was clear at the bottom where we bought our passes. As we ascended the mountain on the chair lift it became foggier and foggier. No biggie we thought, we would take it slowly. What we had forgotten was that it had been a very long time since we had skied a mountain without knowing it at all. At the top therefore non-surprisingly we were completely disorientated. We did not even know if we had to go left or right. A group of not so reckless teens was coming up behind us, they jumped off the lift and powered off to the right. Obviously they knew where they were going, so we followed. 10 seconds later they had disappeared. We could not even see the poles marking the run, we could barely see each other, it was the pitch black equivalent of a foggy day. In good spirits, we started in one direction; Natasja and I following Roland, keeping super close. He took a left and dropped down a small ridge on the right hand side of a pole. I followed a little further to the left and dropped down the same ridge except that, further to the left, the ridge was higher, quite a lot higher. I skied off it and my legs buckled as I landed, because the drop had been greater than I had imagined. It happened in a split second. I landed hard on my left shoulder. It hurt briefly but I picked myself up. We continued down the slope at a snail's pace. Another group passed us. It was the kind of conditions, which make you feel seasick as you ski. The whiteout is so complete your eyes have no way of gauging the ups and downs in the terrain. After picking our way down the slope in a process similar to an army maneuverer, "one," "two," "three," to check we were all still close (Roland did 18 months in the Dutch army, conscription back then,) we made it to a restaurant at the bottom of the hill. We had a coffee, abandoned the idea of going up again and went home. Three weeks later at a Wednesday-morning boot camp training, I raised my hands above my head and felt a click. It did not hurt; it was just uncomfortable. I went home, peeled off my t-shirt and felt another click. I tried a front crawl-swimming stroke and every single time I brought my left hand forward and up, it clicked. I noticed a small bump at the base of my neck, above my sternum. I waited three weeks for it to stop clicking, go down or disappear. It didn't. I visited a trauma surgeon, had an MRI and then he asked me if I had fallen recently. I could not remember any incidence of a fall and then it dawned on me, that stupid episode on the mountain. He confirmed my fears, something was wrong with my shoulder bone; he diagnosed an "unstable clavicle." He said he could do surgery to shave off the end of the bone to make sure that it did not jump in and out. He could offer no guarantees that it would improve the situation and he said there was a risk it could hinder. So on one rainy morning in a doctor's office in Luzern, my triathlon days came to an abrupt close.

However, as hopefully you know by now, "we may be losers, but we are not quitters." So on one rainy morning in Luzern, a mountain trail runner and ultra-marathon runner was born.

GOLD: New dreams, new goals, new people, new experiences AND new equipment…

SILVER:
If you still need to participate in a triathlon, there are always triathlon relay teams.

BRONZE: Be grateful it is nothing more serious.

Part II
MY
TRI SISTERS'
JOURNEY

Training for and taking part in Ironman Switzerland changed me forever. It was, for so many reasons, such a defining experience in my life, that I felt compelled to share it with other women. Take from my Ironman triathlon experience what you wish, you don't have to run an Ironman or even take up exercise but know that if you put your mind to something, you can achieve it; if you really want something it can be yours. This feeling of internal strength still gives me so much energy. With this energy I enjoy life at a higher voltage than before. I see the world with clearer vision; the cup is more than half full. When confronting problems, emotional upheavals and stress, I have greater reserves, I can rely on myself. I went on a journey to get to know myself and I feel I have a special, trusting relationship with myself now. After Ironman Switzerland, I could hardly contain myself. I wrote to the organisers of IRONMAN Switzerland and asked them if I could send a questionnaire to all the female participants. The questionnaire was eventually available in four languages. I wanted to find out if others were experiencing the same high as I was. IRONMAN Switzerland agreed and along with other women who filled out my survey, I received 40 responses. It turns out that many other women had similar experiences. Then I knew I had to share our stories with other women. It was only right that as many women as possible should have the opportunity to push their boundaries and bodies and soar in self-achievement. So this part of the book is a tale of triathlon, of ambition, discipline, drive and some pain. It is our journey, our laughs, and our tears. Once again, these stories, these experiences are written by women, about women, for women. I hope they inspire you. I put my tri-sisters' quotes in italics and prefaced them with a 🏃 or

another icon like 👟 or 🏆 so it is clear that these are responses to the questionnaire. A few are my own tips added under the appropriate heading.

Names of all the IRONMAN Switzerland and the IRONMAN UK participants and others who contributed:

Bianca, South Africa, Clair De M, France, Cykelsilden, Danish, Deborah B, Great Britain, Diana S, The Netherlands, Eve B, USA, Hildi, Great Britain, Ingrid Le T, South Africa, Jessica H, Great Britain, Joanna K, Poland, Karen, Great Britain, Kathrin Z, Germany, Kelly K Belgium, Kirsten S, Denmark, Laura, Great Britain, Lisa M, USA, Lou, Great Britain, Maria W, Sweden, Mariana C, Mexico, Mary Beth, USA, Nadine, Germany, Pat, Great Britain, Rachel, unknown, Sandra F, Switzerland, Sarah, USA, Seonaid, unknown, Sharon, Great Britain, Simone T, Austria and Susanne M, Germany and some who chose to remain anonymous.

Huge thanks to each and every one of you, you all rock x

20: Life changing raw endurance-hear me roar

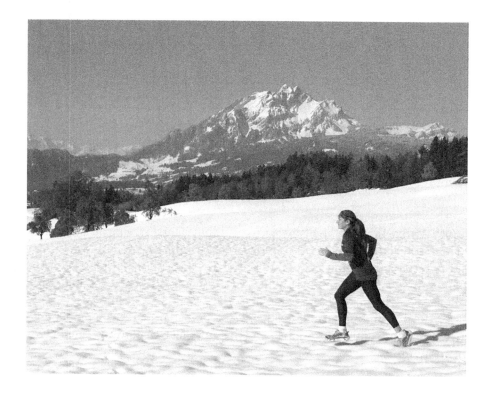

Question posed: "How has participating in an ultra distance triathlon influenced your life?"

Approximately 162,000 women on this planet have completed an ultra distance triathlon. The finishers of IRONMAN Switzerland joined this unique group of women athletes in July 2013. This is what they and the others who answered the survey have to say about how completing their IRONMAN changed their lives.

🏃 Raw endurance like that changes everything.

🏃 I now know that when I put my mind to it, I can achieve anything and I can rely on myself 100%.

🏃 I am proud of myself and admire my body for its performance; I met some really nice people. I have also been asked to coach two acquaintances.

🏃 Healthy, balanced and satisfied life. I have become a much calmer person. More capable of solving every day problems e.g. Stress at work. And I am never sick!

🏃 It takes at least 6 months to train properly and during these months you have to stick to a way of life. You have to know why you do this, and be committed and consistent. It's a choice and a lifestyle.

🏃 It made me more disciplined. Before I was not that disciplined and had difficulties setting and working for goals. Now it is part of my life to work with goals and plan for that.

🏃 Yes, I feel like I need to do it again and feel all the rush and energy of the race. I feel more confident and feel like I can do anything. I feel good about myself, proud of who I am and what I've done. I've rediscovered my competitive side and how much I love sports and training.

🏃 More self-confidence.

🏃 A LOT! Found friends, found confidence in both swimming and biking. And I know that I can achieve something no one thought I could do (I remember my husband strongly advising me to pull out before the first time saying that I simply had not trained enough (rightfully so…)

🏃 I am much stronger now, mentally as well as physically, and don't admit defeat as easily. At my recent annual work appraisal my boss told me that if there were ever a problem we didn't know how to solve, or something we didn't know how to do, I was like a terrier, and would work away, refusing to accept it couldn't be done, and always finding a solution. I think some of that has come from completing IRONMAN Switzerland – or maybe having that mind-set was what made Ironman possible, despite never having ridden on anything other than my childhood BMX when I signed up!

153

🏃 It was really amazing to have completed it and I'll always have that. It was an important day in my life that I always look back on with real satisfaction.

🏃 It has transformed my life. I now know that I can achieve anything. I just have to want it and keep going. When I first told people I wanted to do an Ironman some of them said I couldn't do it, that I wasn't fit enough and, in one particularly memorable instance that I wasn't 'the right body shape'. Then when I DNF'd (did not finish,) my first ultra distance triathlon, I felt terrible, because I was afraid they were right. Then I spent another year training and I became the person I wanted to be. I've applied the lessons I'm learning from Ironman in my career and am pushing through the fear and raising the bar, applying for and getting jobs that I thought I couldn't do or didn't deserve to have before. It's all the same thing; self-esteem, and knowing that you can do anything you want if you just work out what you need to do and go out and do it.

🏃 IRONMAN Switzerland has broadened my goals in life, as well as enhanced the way I live my life now in so many different ways. Before IRONMAN Switzerland, my training events kept me local and limited distance-wise. Since discovering long distance triathlon my events take me all over the world! With the advent of FB, Twitter and Strava/Training Peaks (on-line training programmes,) I am now able to stay in daily contact with athletes from all over the world who compete in long distance triathlon events worldwide. Many of us train together virtually for months leading up to the events, then when race week arrives, we meet face-to-face for the first time and spend time together with our families. We've hosted our European friends when they've come to Florida to compete in events around the state and vice-versa. The summer of 2013 was especially rewarding. A few days after competing in IRONMAN Switzerland, my husband and I drove to northern Germany, stayed with our friends for a few days, then drove to Glucksburg, Germany and competed in the Ostseeman Triathlon the following Sunday. It was an ultra distance race, but my European friends included me in their relay teams and I had the pleasure of running the marathon portion of the event and crossed the finish line with five of the most amazing athletes in the sport!

🏃 My daily life is totally organized around training. Vacations are nearly always spent at a Training Resort. I pay much more attention to my diet and ensure I have enough sleep.
🏃 I always work to improve myself and to become faster, more sport and better diet. I have many new friends with whom I can do sport together.

🏃 It dramatically changed my life. I loved the training and the planning and the organizing of my time. It changed my lifestyle. I am now up early, rarely drink more than a glass or two of wine and eat much healthier. I also plan most of my vacations and travel around races, and spend a lot time with friends that want to run, or bike, and meet for races. When I think about moving to a new city or getting a new job, I think about what training would be like in that city. I also find myself often trying to encourage other people to participate in races, or healthy activities.

🏃 It defines my lifestyle – I also row competitively

🏃 Ultra distance triathlon training is not a hobby but a life style. Often there is little time over at the weekend for other free time activities and even vacations are planned around Training resorts and competitions. Overall the physical effect is all round positive as when I purely ran marathons I had many more injuries. Additionally, I have many new friends and have met many interesting people through long distance triathlon.

🏃 It has also made me realise how important it is to be healthy and train and eat properly. As race day approached I'd been off alcohol for over a month, my training sessions were enjoyable I felt on top of the world. Exercise and eating clean were key in this lifestyle.

21: Can I be an ironwoman? – Why do we do this?

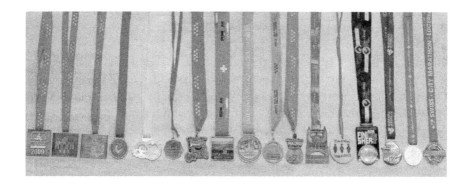

The women who responded to the survey came from 13 different countries. They ranged in age from 27 to 60 at the time of IRONMAN Switzerland. Some had kids, some did not, some were married, some not. Some were in full-time employment, others part-time and others were stay at home mothers. So they were different, but what I was interested in was what they had in common and their characters. In the questionnaire, I asked them to have their best friends describe them in 5 adjectives. Bold type used to indicate words, which came up repeatedly. Here is the list in no particular order:

Intelligent, **determined**, adventurous, open, dedicated, motivated, nuts, strong, enormous willpower, active, happy, willing to try new things, a bit naive, cheerful,

driven, disciplined, outgoing, fun, funny, accomplished, **crazy**, tough, committed, accident-prone, optimistic, positive, energetic, not an ordinary girl, humorous, well-balanced, well-organised, patient, supportive, **positive**, motivating, interested, **stubborn**, understanding, ambitious, lovable, kind, witting, giving, structured, wise, realistic, **brave**, motivated, caring, thoughtful, busy, forward thinking, easily bored, empathetic, loyal, adventurous, good communicator, warm-hearted.

So for comparison's sake I asked my Pilates' friends to do the same exercise, they came up with:

Witty, down to earth, spontaneous, straight forward, good-looking /radiant (because the eye needs pleasing too!) smart, funny, loyal, good mother, beautiful, open-minded, smiling, joker/playful, music lover, lovely, practical, intelligent, sociable, flirtatious, happy, honest, artistic, resourceful/skilful, dedicated, hard-working, generous, caring, trustworthy, diligent, elegant, talented, positive, generous, empathetic, cares for others, hard-working, loving, fun, reliable, discreet.

So there is a difference! Whilst we find fun, loyal, positive, open and happy in both lists, the ironwomen triathletes seem to be crazy, stubborn, brave, determined and driven. We don't find flirtatious, artistic or music-lover. This makes sense of course!

Get a pen and paper and answer the questions below:

How would you describe yourself in 5 adjectives?

1_____

2_____

3_____

4_____

5_____

How would your best friend describe you in 5 adjectives?

1_____

2_____

3_____

4_____

5_____

"What motivated you to take on the ultra distance triathlon challenge?"

So if the question is, "Can I be an ironwoman?" The answer has to start with what makes an ironwoman different to the rest of the population as we saw above. In part it must also be due to what is motivating her to achieve this particular goal.

When posed the question "What motivated you to take on the ultra distance triathlon challenge?"

These are the responses I received from my tri-sisters.

Ironwoman:I read that ironman distance triathletes are highly insecure, always seeking approval. I asked fellow ironman triathletes, they all agreed; we are just continually striving to be better individuals.

Ironwoman:Since I found long distance triathlon, I feel I can tell my children that anything is possible, you just have to try and I feel I have achieved something to be very proud of.

Ironwoman:For the challenge and to prove I can do more than I thought I would ever be able to do.

Ironwoman:I needed a big challenge. I'd done marathons before and a friend of mine advised me to step into triathlon. Almost everybody thought I was nuts when I said I wanted to do an ironman...that challenged me even more.

Ironwoman:I just wanted to prove to myself what I am capable of. I always look for another challenge to achieve.

Ironwoman:I have completed several short and medium distances and decided it was time to take on the challenge of completing a full distance triathlon – always wanting to test my limits.

Ironwoman:To try and achieve something that I previously thought was impossible.

Ironwoman:Sport, Fun, to be an iron(wo)man ☺

Ironwoman:I've always been a sports person, but never thought about doing an ultra distance triathlon until I moved to South Africa and started doing triathlon, where lots of people were doing IRONMAN South Africa and 70.3 (half distance.) My husband always said he wanted to do one and suggested we should plan it for one year after we arrived in SA since there was IRONMAN South Africa held every year. When we moved to South Africa I had to quit my job, so I was struggling with being at home and feeling a bit useless and not having any challenges or accomplishments that made me feel good about myself; I had a lot of free time. When my husband suggested we should train for IRONMAN South Africa, I decided to join a group for training and started a program for 70.3. We had decided to start by doing a 70.3 first and then do the full distance triathlon. At first I only imagined myself doing a 70.3 and would see what happened next. After 3 months of training for 70.3 I was so excited and felt so good, I felt like I was finally doing something worthy, and that I had a challenge again. It was like, although I wasn't working anymore I was still doing something important to be proud of, that's when I decided I HAD to do the ultra distance, I wanted to keep the challenge going, keep feeling good about myself and doing something unique, something that kept me busy and that was making me feel full of energy and satisfaction.

Ironwoman: Enjoying sport, three disciplines instead of just running and above all the question of whether I could really achieve it.

Overcoming physical hurdles drives others. I was astounded to read stories of women completing IRONMAN Switzerland despite having Multiple Sclerosis or asthma and from women who in their early years did not consider themselves athletic at all.

Ironwoman:Some years ago I was diagnosed with Multiple Sclerosis and I wanted to know if I could complete an ultra distance triathlon – on top of that my 40th Birthday was coming up and I thought this is the chance to do something crazy.

Ironwoman:I was asthmatic till the age of 15 and was not able to do sport. I only really started partaking in events when I was 29.

Also celebrating entering into a new decade is quite the motivator.
Ironwoman: Turning 40 was a huge milestone for me. My first challenge at 40 was my first marathon in Berlin, Germany in 2010. My next challenge was the full Ironman in Nice, France in June 2011. I figured if I could conquer these challenges at 40, the rest of my life would be full of more fun challenges!

Age it turns out is not an excuse. To put your years into perspective read "The Grace to Race," by Sister Madonna Buder, otherwise known as the Iron Nun. She started running triathlons at the age of 55, and has completed no less than 45 ironman distance triathlons. She holds the world record for the oldest person (male or female) ever to have done an ironman distance triathlon, finishing the Subaru Ironman Canada in August of 2012 in a the of 16 hours and 32 minutes at the age of 82. Obviously we are not all made of the same stuff as Sister Madonna but age in triathlon is different than age in say sprinting or tennis.

Some come to triathlon as a result of injury. This might be surprising as you might assume that so much time training might cause injury but the three disciplines are easier on the body than one might think. Swimming in particular helps the muscles relax and recuperate.

Ironwoman:I kept getting injured just running, and someone suggested that triathlon might help prevent injury.

Ironwoman:I found a group online called the 'Pirate Ship of Fools' who said that it was possible to go from zero to ironman finisher within a year. It sounded kind of fun, and also kind of nuts, so I signed up for Ironman Switzerland. Then I had to buy a bike, and learn to cycle on roads for the first time – I did the cycling proficiency course that usually school kids do!

Ironwoman: All my life I have been a sportswoman. For 12 years I was training Korfball and when I had a knee injury I was afraid that I'd never be able to do sport again. Then I started running. After two years of running I started to think about triathlon. It was a big challenge and great adventure to me.

Ironwoman:I just wanted to try it on. And I start training. I started my tri challenge with a ½ distance triathlon. I crossed the finish line and I was deeply in love with triathlon. The next step was to participate in and finish a long distance triathlon.

Ironwoman:It just came like this. I have sworn before never to take part in such a crazy race and one day I realised I wanted to do it. Then I got injured during my training and had to transfer my race entry to another event 5 months later. From that point on, I was more motivated than ever before. I had to make it to the race injury free and in the best possible fitness condition.

Some women came to the sport through seeing others participate in an ultra distance triathlon.

Ironwoman: Volunteered at Ironman Lake Placid in 2007 and 2008 and was amazed and wanted to be part of the experience.

Ironwoman:I had been running for about 15 years and had completed a few marathons and numerous shorter distance races. I had also done a few sprint distance triathlons and one half-ironman distance race. One day at work a friend walked into my office and asked if I wanted to train for an ultra tri. I told him no way, he was crazy. I didn't have the time to do it and the weather was going to be too cold during the winter to train. The problem was, the second he mentioned it; I couldn't stop thinking about it. I started researching the different training programs and pretty soon it was all I could think about. Next thing I knew, I was signing up for the Nice, IRONMAN France.

Ironwoman: My friend Jason and I met two amazing Canadians, Leanne and Stuart, when climbing Adam's Peak in Sri Lanka in 2004. They had both done Ironman Canada and I was completely in awe of their achievement. This was the first time I had ever heard of the long distance triathlon and I wanted to do it ever since. At that point I hadn't even done a marathon before. Jason and I have both gone on to do the long distance triathlon.

Ironwoman: Well, I know these 2 crazy ladies that had the idea that they wanted to do an ironman. . I had run since I was 20 years old and knew I was ok at it. I had done 1(!) 100mile Death Valley (close to Las Vegas and VERY hot and dry climate) bike race without really training apart from some km just getting used to having real bike shoes using another friend's bike. The bike I didn't use until the race day). So although I knew I was a bad cyclist I knew I could manage through endurance. What really made me join though (apart from these 2 ladies are really nice and I had a fun social interaction over sport instead of coffee) was that I thought that I could learn to do front-crawl. When we started training I never really thought much of doing an ultra triathlon, I just thought it was fun to train and learn something new with these newfound friends. Crawl was harder than I thought so that made me think that I probably would never make it.

Ironwoman: I have been competing in triathlons for the past 6 years, then I read Chrissie Wellington's book and that motivated me to set my next challenge. My colleague who had already completed one also helped give me the confidence to do it and finish it.

Ironwoman::In 2011 I accompanied my then boyfriend to IRONMAN Lanzarote. After standing, watching on the sidelines for 8 hours I said to my friend Kathi, "I want to do this." In December 2011, I started on my training and completed my first half distance tri in 2012.

And those who are looking for a new lease in life:

Ironwoman: About 7 years ago I dumped a boyfriend and wrote a bucket list, as part of that list I went on a surfing camp in Portugal, there I was introduced to triathletes. When I came back I started with sprint distance and doubled my distance every year, I now average 2 long distance triathlons a year.

In his book, The Triathlete's Training Bible, Joe Friel has a chapter titled, "Assessing Fitness." So to determine if you have an ironwoman in you, look at the Personal Profile and take the fun and interesting "test" and see what comes out of it. The book is an excellent book, possibly the only triathlon book you really need to purchase, except this one of course. There are other similar exercises on-line as well. Contemplate your rational and irrational motivators as defined by Ben Greenfield in chapter 2.

Write them down; just for yourself nobody else need see them. Your rational and irrational motivators:

What are your rational motivations for considering a long distance triathlon?

What are your irrational motivators for considering a long distance triathlon?

_____

_____

_____

_____

_____

_____

_____

_____

22: Treasure trove of our 100's of tried and tested tips to success

12 things
SUCCESSFUL
people do
DIFFERENTLY

1. *They create and pursue focused goals*
2. *They take decisive and immediate action*
3. *They focus on being productive, not being busy*
4. *They make logical, informed decisions*
5. *They avoid the trap of striving to make things perfect*
6. *They work outside their comfort zone*
7. *They keep things simple*
8. *They focus on making small, continuous improvements*
9. *They measure and track their progress*
10. *They maintain a positive attitude as they learn from mistakes*
11. *They spend time with motivational people*
12. *They maintain balance in their lives*

[16] daily quotes

I think we did not really know what we were getting into when we embarked on our triathlon journey. Very soon, it became clear we had a lot to assimilate. Just about each time we went out training we learned something new. In this chapter, I will pass on our new knowledge and also tips from the other Zürich participants. The survey question was, "Name your top three training tips." This list is worth its weight in gold because it is information that would normally take years of experience, successes and failures to accumulate. Here I present a treasure chest full of ironman distance triathlon nuggets. I would have loved to have sat down with all these courageous, wonderful women and share stories. In the survey, I asked each IRONMAN Switzerland participant to share her three top training tips. I sorted them into:

Running,
Biking on the trail
Turbo biking
Biking Technology
The biking mind
General training,
Mental side-mind over matter
Nutrition
Injuries

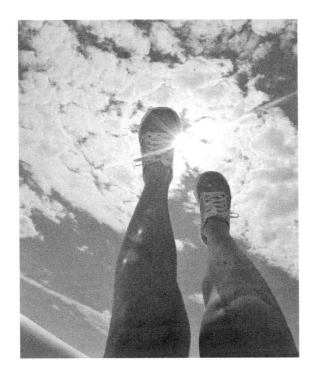

Running:

This one might be my favourite tip of the whole book because it shows such a sense of fun, humour and humility.

🏃 Go heavy partying and then run for 2 hours the next morning: this awful feeling comes close to how you will feel during the running part of an ultra triathlon.

🏃 Run, run, run: Did I mention run? Run as much as you can in your training. Swim and bike are good to know, but running is where you make your time.

🏃 Have an awesome playlist for the run, with music that just makes you feel like pushing it and keeping going.

🥾 I have done at least five 30km sessions watching movies back to back whilst running on a treadmill. I have fallen off it only once so far.

🥾 Test your mind and body by running on tired legs. The day after a 30km go for a 4km run, assuming you are listening to your body and know that it can handle this.

🥾 Vaseline will become your new best friend. You have to stop chafing before it starts, whether it comes from legs rubbing together when running or around the neck from the wet suit. A friend of mine swears by vaselining her feet to protect them from blisters on long runs.

🥾 Run somewhere different occasionally. Just buy a map, find a trail, and bring the enjoyment back.

🥾 Never run more than 3 hours at a time, if your long run would takes you longer than 3 hours, stop at 3 – it takes too long to recover.

🥾 Run the long distance with a group or an organised run.

🥾 Fartlek and the Ladder, your short workout strategies, if you only have say 40 minutes, you can achieve a lot. There is an abundance of these killing sweaty workouts on the Internet. If you don't dread these, they are not horrible enough. Fartlek is interval training, e.g. running 100m fast, 100m walk and repeating 3 times, then next outing 4 times, then 5, building up. The Ladder is running 10 seconds fast, 5 seconds break, 20 seconds fast, 5 seconds break, 30 seconds fast, 5 seconds break, then 20 seconds fast, 5 seconds break, 10 seconds fast, or any combination of up and then down, you can create your own ladder and design your own Fartlek, e.g. using lamp posts on the street.

ADD YOUR OWN:

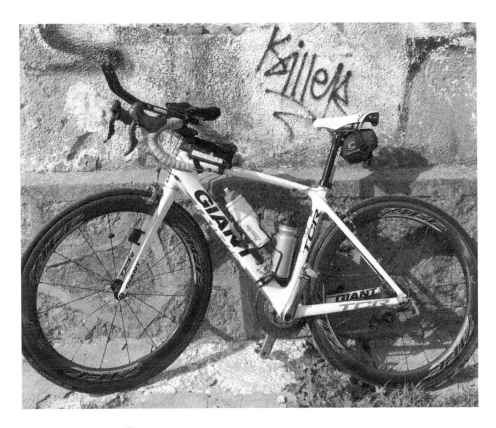

Biking: On the trail:

After each bike you should do jogging to prepare the muscles for the change of discipline, even if it is only a 15-20 minute run, it is very important.

Bike in a group which is stronger and faster than you are but keep motivated; one day you will overtake them.

Spend time on the bike – it will be easier to improve bike time by 5 min than your swimming or running time.

Cycle at least some of the time on your own. Social bike rides are lovely, but on the day of your ultra triathlon, you need to be used to your own company, and able to talk yourself out of bad patches. My first long distance triathlon event was also my first solo cycle ride, and I was kind of lonely on the bike. I ended up singing to myself, and I really can't sing!

Train with and buy a saddle measured to fit your 'sit bones'. Otherwise you will be in agony after 4 hours. Neurofen is very effective too!

We went up a mountain called "Rescafria" which literally translated means Cold Scratch. It was a 10% incline so we allowed ourselves to stop every 2 km, catch our breath and continue. We did this for the entire 14 km ascent. On the descent Kirsten got really cold because at the top we were 1800m above sea level. Halfway down, we enjoyed a big fat cup of coffee, it was delicious, actually I think we had two.

Pay attention to the last few kilometres of a bike or run, when you are tired but happy. One bike ride, Kirsten not concentrating, clipped the side of the pavement and went down. She really hurt her coccyx bone. For a week she was suffering because of a brief lapse in concentration. We swam a lot that week.

Learn about cadence. Track your own using a cadence sensor. These are normally part of the distance measurer on your bike and often have a heart rate monitor too. Read this article for clarification: http://www.active.com/cycling/articles/cycling-cadence-in-training-and-racing. Work for your best average cadence on the bike, this is key.

Experiment using the big cog up hills. The professionals often use the big cog (the crankset, as shown in the diagram in Bike Technology, between the pedals) up shorter inclines. This actually reduces the hardship of climbing. Professionals can do this (and you will learn to do this,) because of their supreme leg strength and mastery of the bike.

ADD YOUR OWN:

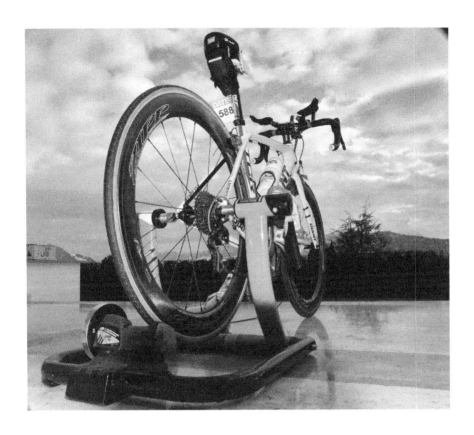

Turbo biking:

🛞 Get yourself a bike stand to turbo at home.

🛞 During the winter get a stack of good DVD's and watch them whilst you train on the stationary bike or on your bike on rollers.

🛞 If you're using the turbo trainer, make it a planned session. Much as I love watching movies on the turbo, if they're good movies you will forget what you're supposed to be doing with your legs!

⊙Take some spin classes and learn different turbo biking techniques. Keep it varied!

⊙When starting a turbo bike session it might take 10 minutes to warm up; get the blood flowing and then the session can begin.

ADD YOUR OWN:

"YOUR PLAN FOR CHANGING A TIRE ON RACE DAY CAN NOT BE…"CALLING A FRIEND" - Race official

Bike Technology:

Have a professional do a proper Bike Fit at least 4 months before your race. You take your bike and all your equipment to a bike shop or someone who has all the equipment to measure you and your bike. S/he will measure distances like feet on pedals to saddle, saddle to handlebars, angle of inclination of your back, width of shoulders and handlebars and tri-bars. S/he will propose optimum distances to ensure that you are not taxing one part of your by straining it unnecessarily. Your body takes enough beating over the 180 km without having to compensate for an easily adjustable seat height or handlebar stem [17]

Take two inner tubes on the bike and get familiar with the amazingly cool blow up cartridges to pump up your tires, time how long it takes to change a tire and you will see how you improve.

Two weeks before the race, we had our bikes serviced. We took them back to the shop where we originally purchased them. After the service, we took them out for one last long bike ride. That gave us time to go back to the store for a second check-up if needed; I had the chain shortened.

Don't worry about how light your bike is, lose weight instead, it's cheaper than a new bike.

Offer help to anyone you might see in trouble. Someone helped me once when I was fiddling by the roadside trying to change an inner tube. Some years later, I did the same for a French guy who was quite shocked that I knew what I was doing.

In the beginning we did not have much idea about our bikes, bike maintenance etc. but we learned! My new Zipp tires were very unreliable when I first received them and I had many flats, so many it was embarrassing. Finally, I took the bike in and they replaced the tires with higher resistance rubber. The problem was solved. BUT we had learned how to change a tire and that was a good feeling. We had learned to carry as many spare inner tubes with us as we could fit into our bike bags and we knew that there were different thicknesses of rubber on tires!

Change tires away from stones or other lose objects, I once caught a stone in tire, got a puncture immediately and had to change the tire again immediately, total amateurs!

ADD YOUR OWN:

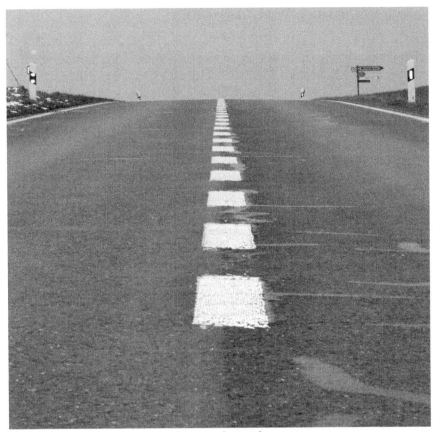
Because, it is a long, long way

The Biking mind:

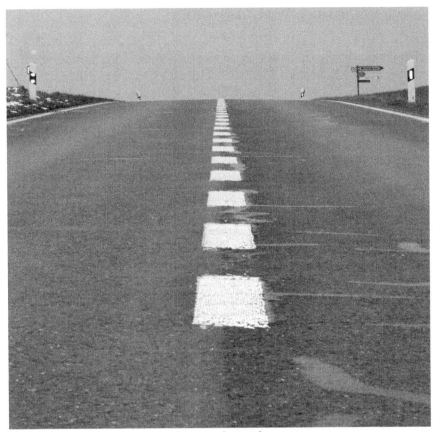Write a book, practice a speech or an important conversation as you bike; the road is a good listener.

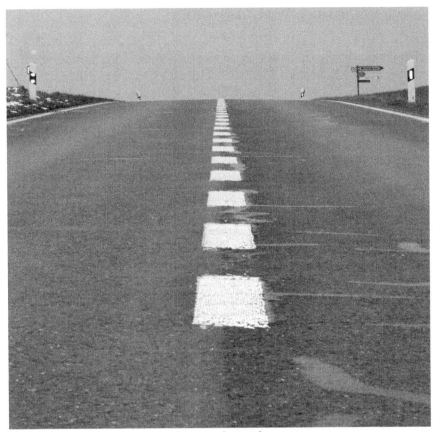Take big yoga breaths on the downhill on the bike, fill the lungs, circulate the oxygen, exchange out the old oxygen for new oxygen. This is knows in yogic talk as

"complete breaths and or 3-part breaths." See: youtube.com/watch?v=S6BGyY7jTX0 or www.yogabasics.com/practice/dirga-pranayama/

A ride that starts slowly can still turn out to be a good ride. Sometimes it can take a while for you to settle down. On a San Pedro outing, I had a flat tire in the first hour and Kirsten was bitten by a wasp (to which she is allergic) so we had to go and find a pharmacy and buy some Claritin. We had covered 30km in 2 hours. We finished a 111 km ride that day in high spirits and full of energy. Certain days will stand out above others as enormously rewarding. Store these in your mind to draw upon when you seem to be fighting yourself. I clearly recall one ride. We arrived at a restaurant in the middle of the Rascafria National Park near the Rascafria Mountain to find the generator was down so we ate two huge white baguettes filled with cheese, eating like that, guilt free is so delicious! We downed a bottle and a half Aquarius each and 1.5 litres of water. White carbs the great invigorator. Then we found our rhythm and that always feels empowering. We felt good even though the wind was trying to spoil the party. It made us feel that the workout was tougher and that our legs were getting stronger. Usually the last 10 km take their toll, as backs, necks and arms stiffen because you know you are reaching the end. Not that day in the mountains, we ruled the bike that day.

Pushing a bike box through an airport is a truly awesome experience. When biking down a hill straighten the more injured leg with tired or pulled muscles so that the muscles can relax briefly. Talk to other people on the bike trail or in the bike store and discover different routes.

Overtake the other cyclists on the bike trails and laugh as they overtake you back.

ADD YOUR OWN:

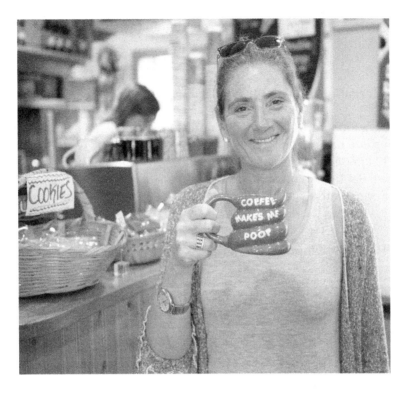

"Coffee makes me poop" mug

General training tips:

👍 Training with your partner, improves your relationship and you learn new things about each other.

👍 Take part in as many competitions as you can and feel your motivation grow!

👍 Don't attempt to catch up lost training units, just continue with the training plan, you will not lose any speed and you will avoid over-training. Work on your weakest discipline, but focus on your strengths, do the sport that you love to remind yourself why you are doing all this training.

 Do alternative trainings such as skating, skiing, Zumba, global training, aerobics. It is a lot of fun, has a good training effect and keeps you motivated. With training you have to be flexible; there will be a sick kid, windy day. We turned back after 32 km one day because it was sailing weather not biking weather. On one ride I had two flat tires on my bike and we took a taxi home. So always have a credit card or money on you.

Learn all the amazing tricks you can do with a Bosu Ball:

Become a Triathlete potty training pro, get that over with first thing in the morning, i.e. work out what makes you go, for me it's coffee!

I do not train kilometre distance, but according to time, my trainer works my overall plan knowing my time allowances. I never run a full marathon distance, and never more than 140km in training, that keeps me motivated and running ;)

For my ultra distance triathlon, I never swam the full 3.8 km, max 2.5 km. On the bike I never did more than 125 km. Take it easy; one should not complete an ironman 5 times during the training phase.

ADD YOUR OWN:

MiNd

---

maTTer

Mental side:

☑ I swim with a dolphin by my side, run with a wolf and ride my bike with an eagle (that motivates me and sometimes helps me overcome my down moments, it sounds a little strange, but it is the mental element.)

☑ Read as much as you can; it will allay your fears.

☑ 8 hours of sleep is more important than getting an extra workout in.

☑ Ignore muscle pain; the muscles can deliver.

☑ Pain is your friend...........really. Get to know and understand your different types of pain. Learn the difference between pushing yourself and hurting yourself.

☑ Its just one foot in front of the other – that's all you need to think about – got me through IRONMAN Lanzarote last year.

☑ Sweat is fat crying – from a friend when I was rubbish at running uphill.

☑ Don't be scared of failing; I have learned more from my 2 DNFs (did not finish,) than my PB (personal best.)

☑ Put up visuals to remind yourself of what you want to accomplish, like race dates. Post your work out schedule where others can see it, and cross off the workouts as you do them. Include pictures of you crossing the finish line of races, super motivating!!

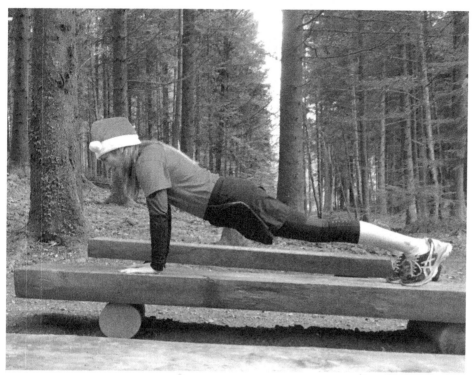

🎄 Even on Christmas Day 🎄

Strength training:

🎄 Do a lot of strength exercises; it is really important to do them in order to avoid injuries during training, but also the race. The stronger you are, the less likely you are to get injured.

🎄 Open up shoulder blades for all disciplines...look up yoga poses to ease the tension in and around your shoulder blades. Use yoga blocks. There is an enormous amount of energy and strength in your upper back just below your neck, learn how to release rather than trap this energy. Talk to a yogi about this.

🎄 Core strength, core strength, core strength. Find a programme and stick to it.

Kick start your core with a 6-week programme and then do core 3 x per week. Check out this website for a great home programme: www.boostingnow.com the results are empowering.

ADD YOUR OWN:

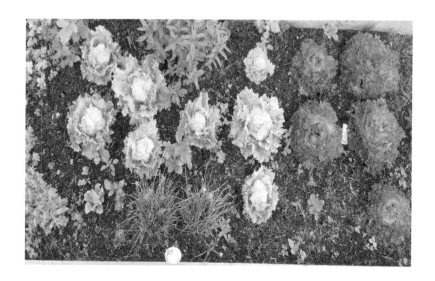

Nutrition:

Have fun when training and make sure you eat and drink lots when you absolve the 4 to 6 hour training sessions.

Eat a lot of protein in your evening meal.

Recovery snack within 30 min after a session actually makes a big difference. I like to have milk w/ chocolate or yogurt.

Vitamin C every day, an orange, mandarin or kiwi to ward off colds. The last thing you want is to get sick with a non-training injury.

Coffee and sugar are a good energy kick. I am not a big fan of sugar in my coffee but if you need energy, it will help!

184

Hydrate especially as it gets warmer, on bike rides we would stop after two hours and drink 1.5 litters of an Aquarius and water mix and set off again with two full bottles. In Spain over 6 hours we might drink 6 to 7 litters.

Learn about sweat, how you sweat and understand the balance of salts, minerals, electrolytes and water. In essence, practice your hydration. Practice your nutrition.

ADD YOUR OWN:

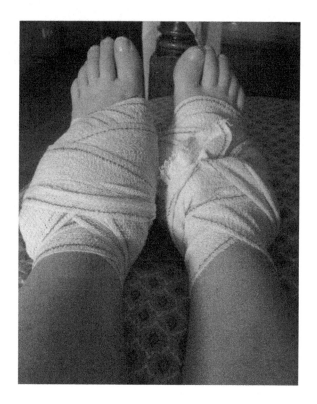

Ice a niggling injury as soon as you feel it. That's ice not swelling under those bandages...

Injuries:

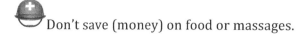Let a professional assess what your physical weaknesses are and get a specific gym programme. Strengthening and balance exercises have helped me to stay injury free.

Don't save (money) on food or massages.

Lots of downtime and enough sleep.

Listen to your body, if your body is telling you to push it, push it hard. If your body says," I've had enough, give it a rest!"

I had hamstring problems for 2 years from just one sprint session, so dumb. I think my hamstring problem came from sprint exercises, so be super attentive to your body when trying something new.

Remember you don't always need to run; we sometimes went on a 10km fast walk, which is fine because you will probably also walk some of the marathon part of that marathon at the end of your ultra distance triathlon.

Trigger point is a type of muscle tension relief exercise. We used to do Trigger Point on Sunday mornings for 40 minutes. (I truly hated those sessions.) Sundays were never long run/bike days I would do those midweek as everyone was at home at the weekends.

Look for improvement in your recovery, specifically in your heart rate, e.g. after a sprint, see how quickly your breathing returns to normal. Record your heart rates so you can track fitness. Also take note of how stiff you might be feeling the day after long training sessions.

Always use heat or ice on stiff muscles, both can be hugely effective. I wrapped ice in Ziploc bag, then in a tea towel and bound it to my injured part using Duck tape, that way I could keep doing whatever I was doing, not training but preparing dinner for example.

My mom had a spa membership so I used to go and have a steam bath after a long run. They were like heaven; sometimes I even fell asleep for five minutes.

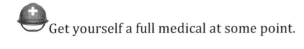Get yourself a full medical at some point.

Even if you have a slight injury, immediately take a break in order to avoid a worse injury and then have to slow down your training plan.

ADD YOUR OWN:

23: Sharpen your pencils-let's make a plan

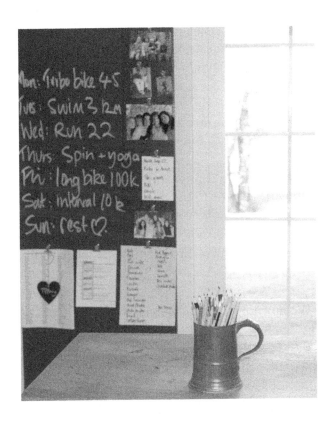

Question posed: "How did you juggle your commitments to fit in your ultra distance triathlon training?"

A commitment to doing either a half or a full ironman distance triathlon means learning a circus skill, the skill of juggling. I think of it as each of our life's commitments/obligations are brightly coloured balls and you cannot afford to drop any one of them. Thus a serious long distance triathlon athlete needs to learn to make a plan and juggle commitments. The plan keeps the balls in the air and the juggling is you being flexible, realistic and armed with clear priorities. Another way of looking at it is keeping all your pencils sharp. This means keeping your life on point and keeping your focus sharp. This was discussed in chapter 4. Here is what the Zürich triathletes wrote about how they juggle their commitments and make their plans. Remember plan in pencil because inevitably plans will change.

Training plan: I think getting a coach is the best thing to do so that you can have a programme adapted to your schedule, travel plans, current shape, objectives... Everyone is different and there are people out there whose job it is to help you perform better.

Get a coach. It can take away the stresses, knowing that you are doing the right training, and don't have to doubt that you're doing enough mileage.

Find ways of integrating your training with your life. E.g. cycle to a friend's house at the weekend or invite your friends to the dam/lake, they can relax while you train, and then you join them for a picnic afterwards.

Plan on Sunday what and when you are to train and where it fits in to life commitments.

Always swam in the morning and afternoons, workouts every second afternoon either running or bike.

I cycled to work, went jogging or swimming at lunchtime and cycled home again

I get up at 4am

Workouts as all other dates (business + private) in the calendar and improvise if necessary.

Waking up very early (4.30am) to fit in my morning session before work. And then an evening session after work. On the weekend I would start early to get the most of the day, so that even with a 5 or 6 h work-out session, I did not miss the day. It takes a lot of organisation and commitment and sometimes you have to say no to social events. But that's a choice and you have to be sure you want to do this and are ready for it.

190

✎With the goal in front of me, there was no way back. Luckily I am quite flexible and got a lot of support from partner, friends and family.

✎My work took second priority. To be honest, I became more selfish. I started saying no to things that I would previously have taken on.

✎When we started training I didn't work so it was very much doing it during the time when the kids were in school and then keeping evenings and weekends free from sports more or less. I started work 3 months before my first Ironman, but it was 3 days a week with very flexible hours, so I could train 2 hours a day without a problem. When doing IRONMAN Switzerland this summer I had started an 8am-5pm job and didn't have my flexible work hours any more. I clearly was not in the same shape (sad how your body deteriorates....) so my 2nd ultra triathlon, IRONMAN Switzerland, was only about finishing and really taking it easy.

✎Commitment of my partner was the most important, to keeping a tight schedule. A personal coach who was "watching me" was critical. It's my kind of way of doing things: when I say I am going to do it, I will do everything to achieve that.

✎As founder of Barrett Court Reporting, dividing up my time as a stenographer, mom and athlete, included a LOT of juggling. My best secret was waking up at 4:30am to complete the time-intensive training, getting the kids off to school by 8:00am, then heading to work around 9:00am. I will tell you that naptime at 4:30pm every afternoon was an essential part of my day. Only 45 minutes of napping, but it was essential.

✎During the build up to my first long distance triathlon, I was self-employed, so it was much easier. Since becoming full time employed, it has been a bit trickier! Swimming happens before work, once a week I run home from work, and also run or use the turbo trainer in the evenings. Luckily my boyfriend also does ultra triathlons and ultra-marathons – so we just meet over big plates of food! Having a slow cooker helps too!

✎The last two months of training it was pretty much training, work and sleep.

I work full-time, so I pretty much gave up most of my social time with friends that didn't involve meeting for a run or ride (on my plan) and was up early to work out, would work all day and usually had an afternoon workout too. The weekends were dedicated to long runs, ride/run or rides. At this time I was dating a professional golfer, so he understood the time it took to train and was supportive of the time commitment and that the time we would spend together was often just at home eating healthy meals and me talking about training. It was not an easy thing to do, but I was very determined to get in all of the training. I would meet friends for dinner, but it would have to be early and I would be the first to leave. I learned to plan and organise all of my time. Even the hour-long commute to work was used to work, answer e-mails, organise meals and shopping lists. I actually think it made me work harder and smarter at work too, as I could not put in the extra hours and had to use every second to the best that I could. I also just did not sleep as much as I used to. Up before 5am every day.

I had to learn not to be so harsh on myself, there was a training programme but sometimes I missed a session the biggest thing was to not beat myself up about it and just say positive for the next session. Training in the morning was also key for me, very few excuses not to do a training session.

As the race came closer my friends and work all knew what I was doing and understood when I said no or when out drinking had a non-alcoholic drink.

24: More aqua phobia-and how we beat it

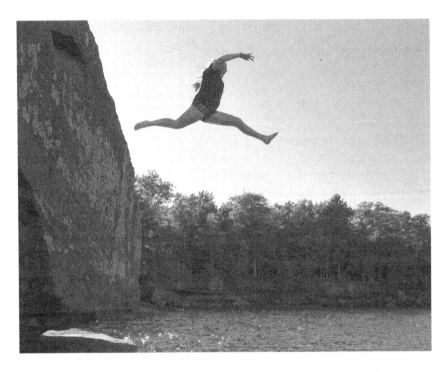

What was that challenge? "Would you jump off a cliff if your best friend told you to?"

Question Posed: Please specify any fears/obstacles experienced during the training and preparation and during the actual race and how you over came these fears."

The answer to this question generated many different responses, but the fear of the swim was by far the most often mentioned fear. There is a lot of fear associated with the swim leg of a triathlon, not just by my tri-sisters but by many triathletes. As is obvious below, the fear takes many different forms. It is the discipline, which often puts other athletes off triathlon. In short, it sorts out the men from the boys. The Zürich women also harboured fears of the swim but managed to overcome them to

complete IRONMAN Switzerland. Below you see first their fears and then their swim tips, how they knocked them on the head.

Swimming Fears:

"South Africa is really famous for its sharks and shark attacks, I always struggled a lot with the open water swims during training, water was sooooo cold and I was just so scared of being attacked by shark, sounds really silly but it was a real challenge for me just to get into the water and train, I just wanted to get out.

I am afraid of getting lost in the lake swim (and often do.)

Swimming, swimming, swimming, the problem for most of us is that you don't get to practice much in the open water.

Did not feel comfortable when swimming, the first few meters were like being in a tumble drier.

I had a fear of swimming 4 km in the ocean.

Swimming has always been the scary part for me, so it requires mental preparation. I learned the hard way (DNF the swim,) that I should not start out fast and get my pulse up – because then it won't come back down again. Swimming training also got to be a bit boring, counting the lanes. I think getting a swim teacher was probably the best thing I invested in, both to learn a better technique and to come up with new ways of swimming in the pool that made it less monotonous.

For me the biggest fear was the swim, I could swim in the open water lake every Saturday but put me in a race and people are knocking me and getting in my way I tend to freak out and have in some smaller races had to be pulled out the water. Having freaked out at an Olympic distance race about 2 months before the big race I opted not to do anymore races (a bold move) but to absolutely get the mileage done in open water and then just remind myself I could do this in the water on race day.

Swimming tips: knocking those fears on the head:

Combine swimming with strength training- this reduces loss of strength and boredom after 2 km of swimming.

Self talk. Just kept telling myself I was going to be fine. Just keep swimming. Calm down. Breathe. Swim your race, you can do this. I also started towards the back and on the side as the people that have done the same race before had suggested.

Swim in an open lake, it is more enjoyable than 76 x 50m.

Practice race specific. E.g. if it's a sea swim, make sure you do enough swimming in the sea, and not just the pool.

Get yourself a swim coach or at the very least 5 swimming lessons.

Find yourself a swimming mantra, something that makes you feel more powerful than the water.

For open water swimming you have to get into open water for training, there is no substitute. Bonus you meet lots of similar people, all mad and very keen to dive into cold water very early in the morning!

Enjoy the healing power of the swim.

➤ On vacation find a local pool and swim there. Variety is good and a new set of swimmers and different conditions help you practice the unknown.

➤ Go swim in a lake with your kids/friends/nieces/nephews in canoes on either side of you, visualise that moment so you can feel them next to you on race day.

➤ Go visit your competition-day lake or sea before you swim it and if possible get in it, meet it, talk to it. Pee in it if you need to, mark your territory.

25: Am I training enough? Am I training too much?

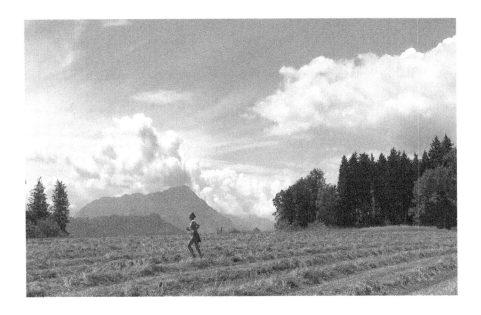

Jumping over the drying grass near home

The question posed: "Please specify any non-swimming fears/obstacles experienced during training and preparation."

Everyone has their own fears and obstacles but the most common answer I received to this question was the constant doubt about the training, was it enough, was it too much, how do I know it will work? Apparently the Zürich finishers trained enough, and not too much, to finish. Here are more of their responses; we all have our hurdles.

You're your demons – 'rinse and repeat' until it is second nature. Go after your weaknesses! I am a really bad descender on the bike, so I did IRONMAN Lanzarote, I am still not perfect but I know I can do it now!

There is always the fear of injury and having to start from the beginning again.

Am I going to finish, will I be able to run a marathon after swimming 3.8km and cycling 180km?

The unreliable Swiss summers were a worry, as they can dampen motivation.

Another Saturday/ Sunday when I had to go out and train instead of staying in bed until 10am

Always asking myself the question, "Why am I doing this to myself?"

Tram tracks (a bad fall two weeks before a World Championship, I now fear crossing tram tracks.)

Will I really be able to complete IRONMAN Switzerland; the distances just feel so crazy far when one is considering a first ultra distance triathlon.

Sometimes the planned training times just did not fit in with my job.

After my stress fracture I was really scared of getting injured again on the running sessions. Any time I had a soreness I was getting paranoid.

4 weeks before the race I fell off the bike. I was injured at my hip and knee. I had problems with running. The last 4 weeks I couldn't run more than 5k. It gave a lot of stress. Also the build of my new TT-bike gave me a lot of stress (f.y.i. it took some time to adjust the saddle to the right height, to be less painful!)

My biggest fear was that the training wasn't working. The first time I trained for a race, I just would start doubting that it was even possible to do an Ironman. Even now, after doing two, it doesn't seem like it is humanly possible to just keep going that long. I realise now that while you have to physically train for the race, so much more of it to be was a mental game. The biggest fear for me is always the fear of not being fit enough and DNF'ing on the day.

I am afraid of being last and embarrassing myself.

26: Don't stop when you are tired, stop when you are done.

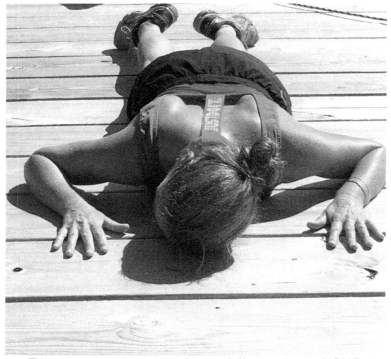

Tabata work out, 6 x 3 minutes full on, all out, DONE

Question posed: "How did you keep motivated during the training period?"

Keeping yourself motivated is part of the mental battle. Not allowing yourself to stop when you are tired but when you have completed the training set for the day or week. This is endurance at its rawest. It is the determined, crazy, stubborn, driven, positive, brave, happy, fun side of endurance. Constantly looking for different training options, strategies to get us out of the door to train is how to keep long distance triathletes motivated. Triathlon training over a longer period of time might mean no biking one week due to weather and a spin class or two instead, more swimming one week due to injury, more running one week as the bike is at the repair shop, it depends on injury, commitments etc. Whatever happens you just have to find ways to keep yourself motivated, and use this variety/flexibility as a motivational tool. This is what my tri-sisters propose:

Always keep the goal firmly in mind. The less you train for an ultra triathlon, the more painful the day will be!

All the time I see my goal. I think that in reality helps to prepare us for the event. This is you realizing your dreams. This motivates me. It motivates the state of mind that I have during and after training, the satisfaction of a job well done.

Daily mental training.

Staying motivated through the training has never been a problem. As a veteran of the U.S. Army, motivation and discipline were instilled at an early age. To me, there is no such thing as skipping workouts or only doing half the training and relying on adrenaline. It's an all-or-nothing attitude in the Barrett household, and it has bided us well through the years. I just set a goal, pick a plan, and follow it through until race day.

It was a personal challenge; therefore I was always motivated. I enjoyed discovering new areas, seeing new sights and cycling different routes. Discovering and understanding the capabilities and limits of my body.

Feedback from people both positive and negative can be your motivation; you build up a mental filing cabinet of people, experience and music that you can draw on when you need a hand.

I was getting faster and faster.

For my first long distance triathlon, it was fear. Fear kept me going I like to dream big. Even if I know I am not going to make it at the first try. I think it's good to set higher objectives than the ones you know you can easily reach. It makes you work stronger and see further and prevents you from becoming lazy.

💪THERE WAS NO WAY BACK... I HAD A DREAM THAT WOULD BECOME REALITY

💪I personally used a lot of motivational videos. I would watch a lot of YouTube videos about Ironman. When I saw all these people pushing their limits I just felt like I couldn't give up, I wanted to push my limits too, I wanted to overcome the pain and see how strong my mind really was, I also wanted to go to that dark place in my mind where you think you may not be able to continue and you just want to give up but decide to just keep going.

💪Affirmations on a regular basis. I made a motivational poster. Watching motivational videos, reading and talking every day about triathlon. Doing alternative trainings such as skating, skiing.

💪Mostly fear, but also excitement. When I signed up a friend told me that your first one is very special, and that I would have a twinkle in my eye for a year, and he was right! And once I'd said I was doing it, people kept asking me about it – I think my work colleagues thought I was mad but brave, and were very encouraging too.

27: "It is amazing how far you can go if someone believes in you."[18]

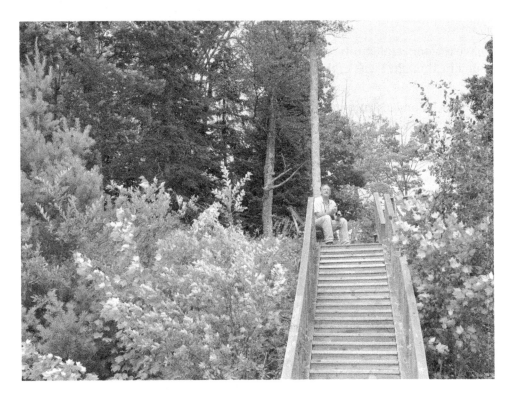

Roland keeping an eye on me as I swam in the lake

Question posed: "How did your family and friends support you?"

Many consider triathlon to be an individual sport. At any level any triathlete has a team around him or her. At the amateur level, this team consists of friends and family. As explained in chapter 11, without my family there would be no triathlon dreams for me. This is how the other Zürich participants commented about their families and their support, responding to the question, "How did your family and friends support you?" Reading the comments below always brings tears to my eyes

👪Sometimes they were a little sceptical but mainly they tried to support me, for example they took over some of my chores, e.g. grocery shopping, cooking and some organising, sometimes they even came to training with me.

👪I have a wonderful family, wonderful parents and partner. They accompanied me occasionally, thought I was crazy but supported me mentally.

👪At competitions my mum and partner are always there. They cheer me on, give me water and gels, and they are very supportive. However, in everyday life my partner gives me the green light on many things. As I began playing with tri, we had a serious conversation about how much time I take out of our lives for a workout. I also asked for a lot of understanding and patience for the period preparing for the competition.

👪Both were massively supportive. I made new friends who became training partners, and old friends and family were great cheerleaders.

👪They were very understanding. The never made me feel guilty when I had no time for them if I had to go on a long bike ride. ☺

👪I'm on a triathlon team and we had about ten people racing IRONMAN Switzerland that year so I had people to train with and support you when you don't think you can do it.

👪Training together with my partner, who would say good and beautiful words, such as "I take off my hat to you," "I am Impressed with your ambition," "you look amazing," these words are inspiring ;)

👪Some join in, the rest think I am nuts, but I have got my mum running at 60 years old!

👪Family and friends were amazing. I was a bit scared of telling my parents, as I knew they'd worry at first, but they're used to it now! And the other 'Pirates' just gently made fun of my accident-prone training and gave lots of good advice about trying to remember to enjoy it! But most supportive of all was my brilliant boyfriend Pete. I had supported him through a 40 hour, 145 mile run the year before, so I guess it was my turn to be the supported one, but he was endlessly patient with my weekly confidence crises, and never wavered in backing me up. I still get goose bumps when I remember seeing him at the final turn into the finishing chute, holding a sign that said 'GO JESS' and looking so proud and happy for me. By the next day he had lost his voice from shouting encouragement, not just at me, but all the other 'Pirates' and fellow competitors!

👪My husband trains and started the race with me. My siblings, parents and friends each run a part of the marathon with me, for support.

👪The best way for them to support me is to accept that I won't always make it to for a dinner or social evening. But then we always manage to find a time to meet and have a chat, even if it's a quick one.

👪They were always there for me. Most of the time I didn't need to cook. I got food and training advice from my partner, as well as massages. Family supported in the sense that they cheered during race day.

👪I took my husband on a "romantic" weekend when we both first tried to bike 180 km. They still joke about that at his work; how his wife arranges these crazily romantic weekends for him :o) As I did most training when kids in school and husband at work the support on a daily basis did not have to be there. But we have always liked to do active stuff and my husband also likes to try new things out, so he started to train for a half distance triathlon and even got a team from his work to do a relay and swim during lunchtime. After completing the first race my kids have been extremely proud talking about their strong ultra tri. mum – which is hopefully also an inspiration to them.

👪My partner and my mother in law kept me from household and garden activities. My boss gave me space and room to work, and be flexible. My friends helped me with advice on food, training etc.

👪Friends and family were just always impressed with the challenge I was about to undertake, their amazement in this challenge kept me going. As did a particular colleague, when I nearly pulled out of the race (twice) we had a little chat and he

205

convinced me again that I should continue and compete in the race. The other 2 things that helped was 1) other people's matter of fact confidence that I would be able to complete it 2) I had encouraged 2 other people to sign on and I couldn't let them down.

👪A lot of my friends are triathletes, so understood. Having said that, I didn't see as much of my family and friends as I wanted to. I'm currently training for IRONMAN Austria in June, and am putting together my 30-week training plan to include scheduling in time to see family and friends.

28: All our race day fears and how we overcame them

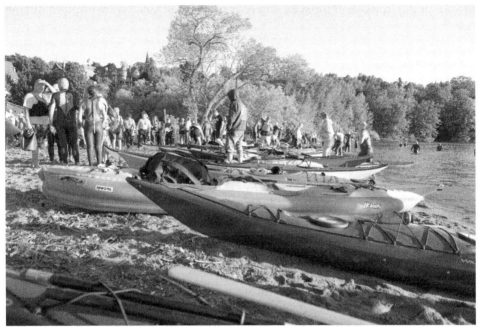
The rescue canoes preparing to launch

"Courage is knowing what not to fear." –Plato

Question posed: "Please specify any more fears/obstacles experienced during the actual race." And "Please specify how you overcame them."

I am fairly certain that every single athlete taking part in an ultra distance triathlon has a list of fears. I asked the Tri sisters to list any fears/ obstacles they experienced during the actual race and how they overcame those fears/obstacles. This is how they responded. First the fear, followed by how they knocked it on the head.

Cramp in the upper calf muscle, and fear of being struck and wounded during the swim start.

I engaged in direct training to the body and not the head. I doubled my intake of Magnesium two weeks before the race. Was unable to eradicate the fear of swim start, the only help was to think positively!

During the competition I worried about getting my tactics right. What is the rate of flow that was not too fast to keep me able to have enough power on the bike and then on the run. Is the food that I have prepared and tested, relevant for today? That I did not eat too much, too little? How will my legs be on the run?

The only way to overcome this is to control, to have a plan.

Did not feel comfortable when swimming, the first few meters were like being in a tumble drier. I tried to find a clear path and swam at my own pace. I had stomach problems on the bike; I did not eat anything other than banana and drank lots of water. At KM 150, several of us received a 5-minute penalty, I was really nervous about the run having stomach problems.

I prayed and begged, it worked and the pains were gone. I believed I could do it and pictured myself crossing the finish line.

Will I manage to survive the swim? If I do will I survive pain free? Is my nutrition plan perfect and will I not suffer from diarrhoea? ? How will my quadriceps feel after 180km on the bike during my first running kilometres? Please no flat tire. Please no panic attack during the swim. What will the weather be like? Will I find my bag at Transition?

I know that I am a good swimmer and I made sure I found myself a good starting position. Given that I was not trying to win, I preferred to swim 20 metres further towards the land than in the middle of the sandwich. Remain well nourished, as I had in training. Mental strength can overpower many thoughts and fears. My upper calf was fine, for a flat tire, I prepared by practicing changing tires. If I experienced panic, I was going to turn on my back and breathe deeply. I was committed now, come rain or shine. All athletes have the same needs as I do, so I followed their way through Transition!

Stomach problems twice this year for the first time – it was soul destroying to know that minutes spent in the Portapotty was minutes from my finish time – that's character building.

Turn a negative into a positive – I did interval runs between Portaloos.

Coughing during the swim, cut wounds on getting out of the water, due to sharp edges (irrational maybe but they were my fears?) Stomach pain whilst on the bike, rain and cold so that I would not be able to feel my fingers and feet.

I will succeed; I have trained so hard for this I will succeed.

Stomach problems.

I tried to divert my thoughts, I concentrated on thinking about other things, e.g. spectators, the next aid station, and the finisher t-shirt, also at the beginning of the bike I did not drink or eat.

Proper nutrition. I ran out of energy twice (once on the bike, once on the run). It was really hot and I didn't get enough food on the bike course. I started to get cramps on the bike and realised that I didn't have any energy left.

I stopped in the shade of the only tree on the road and had something to drink and eat to make it to the next aid station. There I had more food and replenished my bottles and after 5-10 min I was off again and in a much better shape.

Fear of technical problems during the bike race.

Stay focused and let the fear go...if the problem appears you will and can solve it. Don't lose energy by fearing things that might occur. Just go with the flow and be confident.

Swimming has always been the scary part for me, so it is again to mentally prepare PLUS lesson learned the hard way is that I should not start out fast and get my pulse up – then it won't come back down again.

Mental training – not allowing myself to get into that panic mode. Then getting a good swim teacher, that also teaches you techniques. Get a swim teacher who knows about triathlon. You don't need to become super-fast in the water (although that is nice of course), what is important is that you learn to swim so you rest and reserve your energy for the 2 other parts of the triathlon.

I was afraid that I couldn't run out the marathon... but I did...in 4 hours and 40 minutes. Not a very good time, but I made it!

Feared losing control...

FOCUS! In Dutch we say: "blik op oneindig" (focus on infinity?!).

My biggest fear experienced during an actual race was the weather conditions. Living in Florida, one would just naturally assume I'm used to the heat. I train in it and race in it, so one would think my body would acclimate nicely to the heat. WRONG. My swimming is all indoors, my bike and run training sessions are completed during the early, early morning hours to avoid the heat of the day. Although I've completed 95% of the prescribed training for an event, toe up to the line uninjured, I've learned all of it can go right out the window if Mother Nature decides to turn up the heat for the day. The lesson was learned best during the Boston Marathon in 2012. I was completely ready to run a 3:40 for the day. My training was superior to anything I've ever trained for and I felt like a million dollars. As the start gun sounded at 11:00am, the sun was high in the sky and the temperature read 93 degrees Fahrenheit. My legs carried me fast. I was on target for 3:40 at the 15-mile mark when the wheels fell off...and fell off HARD!! At the 16-mile marker, everything turned black and my next memory was sitting on the curbside with medics explaining that they could not get a blood pressure reading or an accurate heart rate. I was taken to the hospital and never got to cross the finish line that day.

The heat factor should be a very large and real fear for many athletes. How did I overcome it? This demon haunts me to this day. One day I will return to Boston and seek my redemption. But the best way I've found to handle the heat since has been to analyse exactly what went wrong and learn how to avoid the same mistakes in the future. Enter Ironman Zurich, Switzerland 2013. The weather reports for the week leading up to the event called for KONA HOT weather!! This was totally unbelievable to me, as Europe is known for milder summers than Florida. An average temperature of 75 degrees on race day is one of the prime factors that lured me to pick this venue/event. 2013 would be the exception to the norm. With predicted temperatures expected to reach 100 degrees Fahrenheit during race day, along with my experience with heat during a race in the past, my new mental tactic and goal would be to finish this race...alive. By the end of the day, I had taken in double my anticipated water intake and salt tablets, kept my heart rate 10bpm above race pace, just barely made bike cut-off, but PR'd (personal record,) my IRONMAN Switzerland marathon time, and crossed the finish line intact and well hydrated. ☺ I defeated my 'heat' demon this day and IRONMAN Switzerland will go down as the race that taught me how to dig deeper than I ever had before on any race day. Mother Nature can truly be the toughest of opponents for any athlete.

When preparing for the race they always talked about nutrition and testing your nutrition during training to avoid tummy issues during the race. I always thought they meant testing the products, not the strategy and amounts. I NEVER tested my strategy during training, I tested the products, not the amounts and frequency I was planning to use in the race. On race day I just had too much sugar, too many gels and too much energy drink, when I was on the bike around 40-50k, my tummy ached so much! I just couldn't stay in the aero position, my stomach was in a lot of pain, like cramps. I was feeling really bad, I got off my bike and just threw up, felt better, but not good. I got back onto the bike and kept on going but the pain came back. This was really messing with my head, I still had 120 k to go and a full marathon ahead of me and I was feeling like hell. I had prepared myself to feel bad, to deal with pain, leg cramps, tiredness, but I hadn't prepared myself for tummy pain. I threw up three more times while riding the bike, this was really getting tougher than what I had planned and for the first time, I started asking myself if I would be able to keep going for 8-9 hr. more feeling like this.

I pulled myself together, and just thought about all the training, and that this was just one of the challenges of the race and I had to overcome it. I came here to feel leg pain and push myself to my physical limits, I'm not there yet, and a tummy pain is not a valid obstacle, so I have to keep going, no matter if it's slow. At first I wasn't sure what was the problem then I just realized that maybe it was the gels. I started cutting back on the gels and sports drink and just drank water. I did this until I started feeling better, around the 120k. I was a bit worried about how cutting back on all my nutrition would affect my performance on the run, but I had to risk it. It worked, and I was able to start the nutrition again at the end of the bike.

I got cramp in my calf and felt very cold in the swim – at one point I was trying to stretch my foot out and it's difficult to swim with your foot at a right angle! On the bike I had to get used to being on my own, and regretted not having trained alone more, and about 90 miles I questioned whether I would be able to finish, it just didn't seem possible.

I gave myself 30 seconds to think about quitting, and have a cry, and then told myself to pull it together. I told myself that the only way I would finish is if I made a commitment to myself that I would do it, and to simply stop thinking any negative thoughts from that point on. Since then my friends often tease me about my 30-second 'Power cry' tactic. Looking back, I think that better fuelling might have prevented the negative thoughts, and the need for a Power cry!

Since I did not live in the area I did not have a chance to ride the course. After one loop, I was not very thrilled at having to do those hills again.

My coach always says just to keep moving forward and that's what I did.

Standing at the water start was terrifying. Looking out at how far I was going to have to swim was just frightening. Plus 2300 people just standing there. The first 10 minutes were awful.

Self talk. Just kept telling myself I was going to be fine. Just keep swimming. Calm down. Breathe. Swim your race, you can do this. I also started towards the back and on the side as the people that have done the same race had suggested.

During the race, I had a fear that something would go wrong with the bike. I don't have enough technical skills to fix even a puncture properly.

I prayed to the cycling gods whenever I heard a rattle on my bike!

Fear of DNF. That's all.

Whatever happens now I just keep going and keep pushing as hard as I can while still staying anaerobic. I do not allow myself to think about the next part of the course, just focus on the stage I'm on (e.g. when swimming, think only about swimming and keep pushing till T1).

The mass swim start.

I arrived a little late at the start and stood at the far right hand side and felt quite relaxed. I found my rhythm. Now I know I can achieve anything even if I think I cannot! That is my mentality.

I had a nice race, but the only thing that didn't work out for me was the race day nutrition. The weather was unexpectedly hot and I didn't want to eat solid, which meant I had too many gels and this caused stomach problems. I knew I had to take on food but each bit made me feel sick.

The run I managed on 1 pretzel and a slice of apple slowly nibbling between feed stations. I'm just a determined stubborn person, and just kept on going. People had faith in me so I had no option! I just need to get on with it and do what I needed to do.

29: Watch out world, I am an Ironwoman – new confidence, more guts

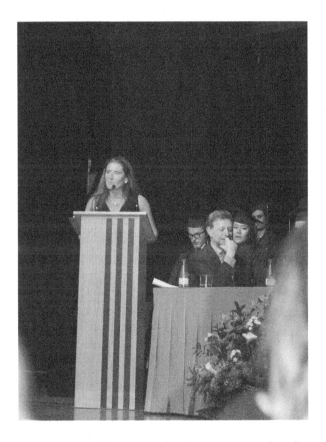

Giving the commencement address at the International College of Spain 2015
Graduation Ceremony

Questions posed: "How did IRONMAN Switzerland change how you perceive
yourself? Has doing an ultra distance triathlon affected your attitude to
life? Has the long distance tri. experience had an impact on your professional
life?"

These three questions, in my opinion, take the rational and irrational motivators discussed earlier, full circle. I loved reading their responses. For me, I am changed forever without a doubt after IRONMAN Switzerland. The week afterwards I was riding a high above the clouds, I was so overwhelmed with myself, my body, it was worth all the training, the stress of preparation and the obsession. I now truly believe I am a stronger person and if I set my mind to most things I can achieve them. There is a very empowering force inside me. This is why I have been so driven to write this book, which turned out to be as much endurance as any long distance triathlon. The other Zürich participants apparently had the same feelings:

Question posed: "How did IRONMAN Switzerland change how you perceive yourself?"

 More self-confidence.

 Able to set a challenge and fulfil it.

 Yes, now I am quite sure that when I undertake something and I work at it daily I can achieve that goal. My family and friends used to say, "you can achieve whatever you want, whatever you put into your head you can pull off." Those were unconscious goals, things, which I did not really control. However in order to finish an IRONMAN, you have to work at it very deliberately and consciously. I have got to know my body, and I somewhat shocked that it has taken me 30 years to achieve that.

 Perhaps more ambitious and focussed on my goal!

🏆 Increased self-confidence because I like my body better. One does not do an IRONMAN race one becomes an IRONMAN.

🏆 Recognition and respect from friends and colleagues.

🏆 It makes me more confident about my abilities. I still have a lot of work to do but you realise that you can be better. It takes time and hard work but eventually you can make it. It also makes you stronger whenever you have to overcome an obstacle in your life.

🏆 I know now that everything/much is possible if you really want to go for it…Not only in sports but in life as well…and if sometimes it doesn't work out like you planned, you still tried it and you will not give up that easily.

🏆 I had never thought of it that way – but a lot of men (I think less women understand what an Ironman really means) really get impressed and I think by hearing others being impressed I have become proud of what I have achieved.

🏆 I'm proud that I can say that, IRONMAN Switzerland, YES I did that!!!

🏆 Before my ultra distance triathlon, I was always 'content' with my role as a mother/wife/stenographer. Life has always been good to me. But once I started running, then swimming and biking, the way I viewed myself definitely turned around. Suddenly things made more sense. My time management skills emerged and the days seemed longer. My self-confidence, self-esteem and self-worth rose to a new level, and my expectations of my capabilities were limitless.

The best part of the journey has been what IRONMAN Switzerland has done for my relationship with my husband. My husband has always loved me immensely, but with the introduction of sports in our life, he has stepped up in our team and taken on the impressive role of logistics manager. And there is absolutely no way I could partake in any event without his assistance. Jim makes sure the training time is set aside each day on my calendar, cooks my meals and prepares my snacks during the day, makes sure I have all the necessary equipment to train and race, registers the family for our different events, packs our bags for trips around the country and world before our departure, organises our transition bags...the list goes on. He is our number one supporter and this allows the kids and me to truly enjoy the various events in which we participate.

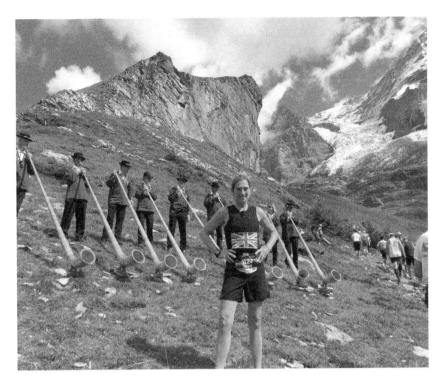

Jungfrau mountain marathon, September 2017, now I can take on any challenge, well at least I will start it ;)

Question posed: "Has doing an ultra distance triathlon affected your attitude to life?"

 Life style wise I have changed but this attitude to life I have always had.

 If you really want to do it you can...

🏆 Live your dream.

🏆 No, but certainly I look at nutrition differently now.

🏆 I have a greater appetite for life with a better standard of living and expectations.

🏆 Everything is possible.

🏆 You don't have anything for free. If you want to achieve something it you have to work hard for it. It's true for long distance triathlon but for anything (work, learning a new language, a new sport, how to play a instrument) I was stubborn before but I think I am even more now. Just don't give up, whatever it takes.

🏆 I know I am now much strong than I thought before.

🏆 No not really. BUT it has definitely given me many, many happy memories that I don't think I would have gotten otherwise.

🏆 Everything is possible with the right FOCUS and good motivation.

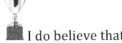 IRONMAN Switzerland has affected my attitude to life. Hitting 40 is never easy for anyone, especially women. My sporting hobby really started at age 39, and by 40, the goals were getting bigger and bigger. Life at 40 has been truly spectacular! As I tackle each challenge and overcome my fears, my zest for life improves. Although every event has not been a success as I've experienced setbacks and failures, I have learned many new things about myself. I have learned that getting right back in the saddle, make necessary adjustments and moving on is really quite easy. My many new friends have encouraged me every step of the way. No longer a cynic, I see the glass 'half full' and accept new challenges with vigour. In the past, I may have found excuses to shy away from obstacles, but today, I embrace them. I may not be the fastest or the best, but I certainly have a lot of fun. There are a few new lines on my face in my 40's, but I know that's from a LOT of smiling, and they're totally worth it.

Today I believe that training your body is also training your mind, your soul. That no matter how difficult the task is; it is accomplishable if you really want it and fight for it. That you may not always be prepared for what's coming, so you always have to be willing to risk it, change the plan and take chances in order to overcome the obstacles.

I'm a lot less prone to depression and negativity now than I was. It still creeps in sometimes, but going out for a run usually clears the mood away. Amongst our triathlon group, we have awards which we give out, and at 2 of my 3 Ironman races I've been named 'Smiliest Pirate' which is probably my proudest triathlon achievement – I'm not fast, and I'm not going to win, but I can make sure I'm having the most fun!

It has made me feel better about life. I feel like with proper training, anyone could do this. I feel like I am more positive in a lot of ways.

I do believe that I can achieve anything I put my mind to.

221

Question posed: "Has the long distance tri. experience had an impact on your professional life?"

I gave up my dream job in order to be able to train for long distance triathlons. Practicing my dream job would have meant training for IRONMAN Switzerland would have been impossible.

My colleagues respect me and admire me for my achievement.

I have become more ambitious and can define things better, (which makes sense because I am much more efficient.) I can listen more effectively and therefore serve my clients more effectively.

They are on my CV, my managers think I am nut but it had made me a more dependable team player, if they know that is how I apply myself in my free time they know that is what I can do at work. I am self-employed, I do contract work, my current contract has been going strong for 3 years, all my colleagues know.

Maybe I need a job where I can work a little less ;)

No, I continue to pursue the same ambitious goals as before and was not prepared to work part-time or "just for the money" anyway. I think it is important that one has can dedicate time equally to other areas of life, not just a job, it is important to separate free time, sport and work.

I kind of have the same attitude at work that I do when I train. I do research and it rarely works at the first try. So I keep working and try not to give up easily – Eventually it's gonna work, isn't it?

NO, I wouldn't say it has impacted how I do my work or how my colleagues and I interact professionally. But when we discuss training and sports in the canteen they

222

are impressed by what I have achieved, and rumours have spread and people I haven't talked Ironman to come up and want to talk about it (again mainly male interest in the sport.)

I became more decisive and disciplined. As a project leader; mandatory skills.

I would say the reverse is true in this instance. My professional life has made an impact on my Ironman experience. As a court reporter, I am fortunate to work with attorneys every day. Attorneys are some of the most driven, ambitious, adventure-seeking people in the world. Many of my clients are triathletes and runners and they travel the world competing in events. One Monday morning in September of 2009, while sitting in depositions, one of the female attorneys arrived slightly behind schedule. She had a great excuse, though. Evidently she had JUST returned from Berlin, Germany having run the Berlin Marathon two days prior. Completely awe-struck by this feat, and the by the fact that she could even walk, my mind wandered the rest of the day. It's all I could think about...maybe this should be my 40th birthday gift to myself – run my first marathon! As soon as I got home, my husband could tell something was different about me. He says I had that 'look' of determination on my face. We ran to the home office and immediately signed up for the Berlin Marathon in 2010. Not only did I run my first marathon in Berlin the following year, my attorney friend ran it with me, also. She has been a constant source of inspiration the last three years as her goals get larger each year. Running is my true passion, but in early 2010, another one of my attorney friends introduced me to triathlon. He felt my running skills were very good, but wanted me to challenge myself a little more. He talked me into participating in my first triathlon in February of 2010. It was hell. I'm not a swimmer and the bike is just plain hard. Although it was the most difficult event at the time, my friend waited patiently for me at the finish line and cheered for me like I was a pro. ☺ This attorney friend introduced me to a whole new world, and we have competed in many events together since. The man that shared the world of Ironman is another one of my attorney clients. In 2008, he was busy training for IMFL. The year was filled with stories of intense training sessions, the victories and defeats. The ease with which he managed IM training as a busy trial attorney with four small children at home simply amazed me. He was the master of juggling a crazy time schedule. A relatively small athlete, standing approximately 5', 6" and weighing approximately 150 pounds, he was a very lean force to be reckoned with. I particularly remember one occasion while attending a trial together last summer in Bradenton, Florida. It was a two-week trial and he was in the throes of peak training. We went to lunch together several times during the trial and that was the first time I had ever watched someone consume plates and plates of food with ease. By the afternoon, the fatigue would set in hard, but he pushed through and assisted his partner to a successful verdict. He went on to complete IMFL (Ironman Florida,) with a fantastic time. As he reminisced about race day in the months following the event, I couldn't help but notice the large smile that always accompanied the story, the glint in his eyes and the enthusiasm it evoked. A very conservative gentleman, he wasted no time acquiring the M-Dot tattoo shortly thereafter and proudly shows it off when he tells the story. As a marathoner and triathlete, his enthusiasm for such a HUGE endeavour was infectious. He inspired me to go for it. In the summer of 2010, I set my sights on Ironman Nice, France and pursued it through the finish line.

My clients are inspirational and support me through it all. I have competed in many, many events WITH my clients – sometimes even on teams with them! We have conquered Tough Mudder in Ragnar, Tennessee, triathlons and running events together! ☺ When your professional life and adventure life come together, it is then you realise just how much of a team you really are. Work is not considered 'work' anymore. It's a profession that brings me much pleasure…and supports future ventures.

Only in the sense that I would love to open a business specialised in triathlon and professional training for triathletes, I've found that sports is really my passion and would love to research about, nutrition, racing techniques etc.

My colleagues think I'm bonkers, but at the same time I think they also admire what I've done. Some of them are even starting to run and cycle, and I organised some of them to do a trail marathon with me as a relay team, which was a lot of fun, and also great team building! At a recent company conference I convinced some of my international colleagues and the owner of our company that running through the boggy Scottish highlands was the perfect post-whiskey tasting hangover cure, and I don't think I'd have had the confidence to be so forward without Ironman! Also, as mentioned earlier, it gives you the determination to carry on, and solve any problem, work out any issue, that in work, as in Ironman, you've just got to get through the bad patch and the finish line is coming right up.

I have more of a balanced life now; I think that helps me professionally.

I feel like after/during the training for IRONMAN Switzerland, I had to become more organised with my time, which made me better at work and in the rest of my life. I also think getting up and training before work helped me get more accomplished at work because I stared off the day feeling like I had already accomplished something.

Somewhat, I will try to apply the same focus I manage in sport to every day activities and my professional life.

I go for jobs that I wouldn't have dreamed of going for before IRONMAN Switzerland. And I get them! I work in an environment where competition and challenges are everywhere. Telling people you did an ultra distance triathlon gives something to talk about, breaks the ice and connects with people, either as they are keen athletes (whatever sport) or they want to start (and I'm a good example of someone who was not fit at school and hated P.E. (Physical Education.)

30: Favourite events, throwing up on race officials, fire ants and other funny stories

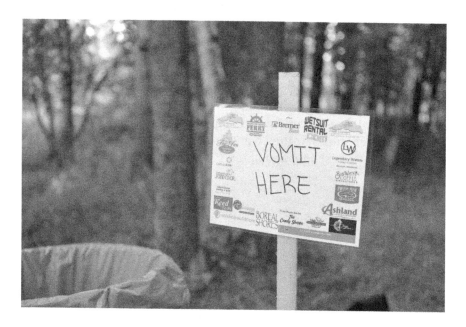

Sign at the Point to la Pointe swim finish

Questions posed: "Name the most fun swim, bike, run, duathlon or triathlon experience in which you have participated and why it was so unique? And add any other funny stories you would like to share."

I wish I had had the opportunity to meet the wonderful women who have contributed to this book. They all have such powerful stories to tell. Here are some of the other adventures, which they submitted in response to the most fun bike, run, duathlon or triathlon in which you have participated question, ones to pin on the to-do board.

Ironman Hawaii. Ironman Hawaii. You hear so much about Hawaii, which may or may not be true, but the atmosphere at Ironman Hawaii really gets under your skin.

Comrades Marathon 89.9 km in South Africa 1997 – I was living in the Comors and was 29 and decided that I wanted to run the Comrades, it was my 30th birthday present to myself (the route passes my parents farm in South Africa and I had been a spectator on several occasions) It was my first race and I won a car in the lucky draw, Nelson Mandela handed me the key. That was the beginning!

2013 in Klagenfurt, during the marathon at the 30 km mark running next to my father and he showed me how proud he was of me and of course crossing the finish line.

Completing my 3.8km swim in my first long distance triathlon in 1.16 was very emotional.

Midnight Man in Kent England, its overnight – and challenges your preparation.

The Trans Vorarlberg in Austria. I thought I would never make the 100km biking at the 2000metres altitude, but I made it!

Participating in the Alpenbrevet in 2013. I had never rode my bike at such a high altitude, with such beautiful views.

Eleven Global Cape Town in 2102. I had a very good swim (swimming straight for once!) and then I just did everything I wanted to do. All the times I put together on a sheet of paper before the race were achieved and it was a great satisfaction at the end of the day!

IRONMAN Switzerland...Because it was the full distance, the scenery was so gorgeous, the weather was hot, which made it even more heroic...the crowd was just wonderful.

IRONMAN Switzerland – as I saw it, it was the "grand finale" of what my 2 friends and I had been training 2 years for. Having us finishing together was special. _Then I would say our first bike rides before we really knew anything about biking - We were falling off the bikes - asking for directions, coming in sweaty and stinky into very Spanish cafés where they looked at us women as if we were from the moon. It was kind of a nice change to the quite posh environment we otherwise moved around in. Of course finishing the swimming part in both my long distance triathlons– the first one doing breast stroke most of the way just not to direction, the second one w/o a wetsuit. That kind of accomplishment made me so happy that the rest of the EXTREME MAN, I felt like I could do it – because the scary part was over.

🏊 IRONMAN Switzerland, my first ultra distance triathlon on 28 July 2013 in Zürich. Never thought I was capable of doing this.

🏊 There are SOOOO many events that have absolutely been memorable, but Ragnar Tennessee tops my list to date. Ragnar is a 200-mile running relay. There are 12 members on the team and each member runs three separate times to cover 200 miles in 36 hours from Chattanooga to Nashville. We ran from early morning, through the night and into the next afternoon. We rented two 12-passenger vans to carry the two separate groups of six. We live in Florida, so we drove as an entire team to the start line for this event, Chattanooga, Tennessee. It's a 14-hour drive. Once we arrived, we stayed on board a renovated antique paddleboat for the night. A serious highlight. During the run, the only sleep you can get for the 36 hours is in the van itself. The tight quarters mean you have to really get close with your friends in the van. Nothing is secret and that's what makes it fun AND funny. We worked together as a team and completed the 200-mile run with no injuries and lots of laughs. The post-finish party in Nashville, Tennessee lasted for the next 48 hours, then we drove the 14 hours back to Florida. Good times. ☺ (We are signed up to do it again next year.)

🏊 Cape Town Argus Cycle in South Africa. Beautiful scenery, lots of people, lots of cheering, an amazing ambience, the whole city is closed and everyone is outside watching the race, 30,000 people of all backgrounds, of all fitness racing, an amazing route, everyone cheering, it was incredible and unforgettable.

🏊 The year after I finished my first ultra distance triathlon at IRONMAN Switzerland, my boyfriend signed up to do one too. The catch was that he had never ever learnt how to swim as a child, so in a year, he had to beat his lifelong fear of water, learn how to swim, and get round 3.8km! He's a good cyclist and runner though, and it was a wave start, so even though he was one of the last out of the swim, he caught me on the run, and we finished within ten minutes of each other, which meant that we have a great photo of us at the finish, both very sweaty, very smelly, and very happy! It makes me smile every time I look at it.

➤ Tough one. IRONMAN Switzerland may be it. It was my first IRONMAN, it was in Zurich, I did it with friends and it was fun seeing everyone on the run. I had the opportunity to go to the Tour de France after the race and that was amazing.

➤ It was definitely my first IRONMAN France in Nice. The bike course was a killer and the day before we had driven the course and I could not believe what we were going to have to do. During the whole ride, I just kept telling myself that as soon as I got off the bike, I knew I would be able to finish the race. So, when I finally came to the end of the bike ride and saw my boyfriend cheering for me it was an amazing feeling. I was all smiles during the marathon and it was awesome to see my friends who had scattered themselves up and down the run course. When I hit the 40 km mark I remember thinking, I am really going to do this. I could hardly believe it. And, running through the finish line and hearing them say that I was an Ironman, it still gives me the chills to watch the video.

➤ Looking at Lake Zürich-it is possible to describe the overwhelming feeling of happiness, knowing that I swam it.

➤ IRONMAN Switzerland, especially watching the little Spanish boy who ran next to his father; motivating him all the time.

➤ IRONMAN Switzerland 2013 was the most fun triathlon I have ever done. I got lost in the lake, and was the 10th out of the water; almost choked to death on the Neurofen foil wrapper, popping a pill at mile 1 on the bike; thought I was lost on the bike course because no-one else was with me for approx. 2 hours; rode on the wrong side of the road because I forgot I wasn't in Britain; got whipped to within an inch of my life by puppy-sized hailstones; and at mile 24 of the marathon pooed in my trisuit because I had just downed a potent Red Bull shot and was unable to hold it in, and at 10pm at night all the Portaloos on the run route were being locked. Thankfully the tri-suit kept it all in. And I made it across the finish line with 35 minutes before the cut-off. One of the physically and mentally hardest and most incredible days of my life.

➤ I did a super sprint tri woman-only race a couple of years ago, what made it fun was I was encouraging a group of 4 friends who were competing in their first race. The fun started at training sessions, getting into the open water with 2 of them as they moaned and groaned about the gooey squelch between their toes. And on race day cycling and running next to my friend and encouraging her to take on the person in-front, we were going to beat her, then the next and the next person we also shared a few Percy pigs as I shouted not time for pigs..... !!

One time I threw up in the Bike Gear Bag that a friendly helper had just unpacked for me. That particular swim made me very seasick!

If you are not a pro, do not take it too seriously, enjoy every moment and enjoy your fellow participants (they have and will go through the same highs and lows as you.)

Sport has opened many doors for me in my life and enabled me to make awesome friends. I have met very interesting people from all parts of the world. It has bought a balance to my life and enables me to do my job professionally.

Sometimes I ask myself if all this is a cry for attention, this is why we torture ourselves so much, then I look at my life in seconds and realize that I have enough recognition and attention, but maybe somehow that is something to do with this. But one memory is there, after I had checked in for IRONMAN Klagenfurt, a friend and I went to eat. My sister, my team leader, left us standing at the reception, she said she had to go and check on something. When I arrived in the restaurant, I could not believe my eyes, my parents were standing at the buffet, it was such a wonderful surprise. I was so happy; their presence was so inspiring. I love it when they stand and cheer on the course wearing their Fan clothing. It is very touching.

Nothing specific, there are a few: I have cried on the swim, fallen asleep running and seen people at their best and worst – to share the experience with 2000 other people is very special. I can't watch an IM on TV without getting emotional.

Bring on the next season!!!

After the swim on my first ultra distance triathlon, I took off my timing chip and set it down whilst I pulled on my socks. A zealous helper threw my wetsuit and chip into my transition bag and threw it on the transition truck. Passing over the timing mat on the way to pick up my bike I noticed that it was missing and ran back to the truck. The volunteers had to dig into the pile of hundreds of transition bags in order to find my bag. It seemed to me like it took hours. The volunteer who had packed the chip was so embarrassed. I reminded him that I was not going to win, and to take his time, as long as I can continue everything was fine.

When I read the "menu" for IRONMAN Switzerland last year I saw they had bouillon and I thought, "Why would they have that?" I forgot about it... until race day. At about 22 km on the run I wasn't feeling great. It was HOT, I was starting to get dizzy and nauseous, I was sick of eating gels and drinking sport drinks. So I decided to grab of cup of bouillon – a nice lucky warm salty bouillon. It was the best thing I could have dreamt of. It was so pleasant to have something that tasted different and it did a good job against nausea as well. I had a couple of more cups at the next aid stations. Until you race you don't know what drinking a cup of bouillon can be like. Now I know it's almost heaven, as weird as it can sound!

Even with a screw in my knee (surgery when I was 17 years old caused by an injury when playing handball) it never stopped me in my way of training for a big goal like a marathon, a bike race or an ultra distance tri.

My funniest story to date goes back to the Citrus Trail Marathon in 2012. Set in the forest of the Withlacoochee State Park in Florida, there's a lot of hills, sand, pine needles and pinecones. The interesting part of the trail marathons is you rarely see a Port-o-Potty. Along my 26.2-mile journey, I had taken in a little too much water and needed to stop for a quick break. It was Mile 24 and my legs were weary, so I decided that 'leaning' against a tree would make things a little easier during my 'pee' break. It was an ever-so-brief break, but as I yanked my shorts up to continue my run, I noticed something didn't feel quite right. Not even a few steps into the run, an excruciatingly hot, painful sensation ran down from my buttocks all the way down the back of my legs. I recognized this all-too-familiar sensation – the bite of the evil FIRE ANTS! Luckily there was no one on this particular stretch of the forest path, so I yanked my shorts down quickly and commenced senselessly slapping my own bottom wildly while running. I'm sure I looked incredibly silly, but this was my instant reaction to the pain. As I pulled my shorts back up and started to run again, the sensation came in another wave. Oh, dear lord, not again! Once again, I yanked my shorts down and slapped my bottom, as well as the shorts. The pain lasted the last 2.2 miles and it came in waves. But, as fate would have it, I was the first overall female across the finish line. I received much swag that morning and it was such a memorable day. Unfortunately, as the day wore on, the welts on my bottom grew. They were extremely painful and lasted for over three weeks. Lesson Learned: Never lean against a tree in the woods, as its 'bark' can be just as bad as its 'bite.'

I won a half distance triathlon race where there were only two women entered! It was really funny as the course was also where some fellow racers were doing a Deca-iron distance (20 times as far as I was) and it made me laugh when these really impressive endurance athletes were very kindly congratulating me and clapping for me – I felt quite embarrassed and not really deserving compared to what they were achieving! But I got a big shiny trophy for it, and it was the first time I'd won anything since an obstacle race when I was about 6.

On another occasion, I was doing a half distance tri to test my kit before Switzerland, and it was three days after my big car crash. So I was quite sore, had a lot of physio tape on me, and I could only breathe to one side on the swim, and was struggling on the run. I got chatting to an older gentleman and we were comparing our excuses as to why we were having a tough day but were determined to finish anyway. I mentioned my car crash, and that I'd been ill for 8 weeks previous to that, and thought my excuse was pretty good. He then told me that he'd had a hip replaced ten weeks before! I guess he won the excuses game!

We did a preview ride of the bike course in Nice, during the ride my aunt got car sick with all the hills and turns, no one was even talking until I finally said, are you guys seeing this! Then my boyfriend and I dropped off my aunt and mom and picked up a girl friend of mine and I guess it was all too much for the car. Because as we were driving back to the house we rented, the car caught on fire. We didn't even notice we were all so stressed out. Then this guy just started pounding on the window. I was such a mess that my boyfriend sent my friend and me to walk the rest of the way and he was left to handle the burning car. He didn't say it to me, but after the swim the next day, he told everyone else that there was no way any of us, there were three of us racing, would be able to do the bike course. He was shocked, amazed and impressed that all three of us did it. And the marathon after...

Believe in yourself and let the others do the talking.

On my first IRONMAN UK (Bolton DNF) I was such an inexperienced swimmer that I exhausted myself in the swim and ended up stopping in the lake and hanging onto a buoy to recover. Then I was so tired that I got lost on the bike and ended up having to get off the bike and walk back down the finish chute because I'd missed my turning and had to do another lap of the course. Needless to say, I didn't make it and the broom wagon picked me up...

232

Also, I collapse and throw up after every full distance triathlon. It's tradition. I am aiming to get to the end of one and being able to walk away from it, rather than crawling.

Two things that got me through the race and became our motto…. 1) I read an article about a month before the race saying the oldest UK female ironwoman was 71, the motto then became if a 71 year old can do it, so can I! 2) Race day was expecting extreme weather conditions and the wetsuit was banned. As we sat in the boiling hot tent at the pre-race presentation, realizing that it was too late to worry about the wetsuit or our training plan or anything else – we realized the race would be what it would be and we would be ready to race it, thus our motto became – it is what it is.

ADD YOUR OWN…………

APPENDIX A: THE LIST WE MADE FOR MARIA FOR EXTEME MAN
SALOU

Swimming:
Earplugs
Flip-flops
Wetsuit
Two caps
Two Goggles
Waterproof Sun lotion
Tri watch
Tri/Swimsuit
Towel
Lollipop (for after swim to get rid of salty mouth)
Aspirin
Water and energy drink
Energy bar
Footbath and a bottle of water for filling the footbath
Vaseline
Tissues
Eight-hour cream
Ginger (in case of feeling sea sick)

Biking:
Chapstick
sandwich
Helmet
Socks
Gels and energy bars - nothing that melts
Tape (to attach energy bars to the bike)
Gloves
Water and energy drink
Shorts and bike shirt

Vaseline
Sports bra
Sun lotion
Sunglasses
Aspirin
Proper pump
Arm warmers and leg warmers
Phone Money
Toolkit
Gas refills (for speedy inner tube inflation)
Spare inner tubes
Extra water and energy drink

Running:
Towel
Underwear
Shorts Sports bra Sun lotion Socks + long socks
(Music) – check if allowed in race
Cap
T-shirt
Gels and energy bars
T-shirt with long sleeves
Blister plasters
Headache tablets
Watch?
Money
Running shoes
Hair elastics

After the race:
Sweatshirt
Sandwich
Other shoes?

DEFINITELY DON'T FORGET: Id and registration

APPENDIX B: MY TIPS ON HOW TO LOSE THOSE EXCESS KILOS/POUNDS TO GET TO YOUR DESIRED RACE DAY WEIGHT:

1)   Margaret Webb in her book "Older, Stronger, Stronger" talks about eating a "wheel-barrow" load of vegetables. Just about any vegetable is good and raw is better.
2)   Reach for fresh vegetables over fruit. Lunch and dinner are a festival of raw vegetables.
3)   Put lots of colour on your plate, I don't mean 50 shades of green, different colours: beetroot, carrots, tomatoes, sweet potato, peas, spinach, corn, cucumbers, yams, kale, peppers, aubergine, cabbage, white/green asparagus, chillis, pumpkin, mushrooms, courgettes, endives, Brussels sprouts, squashes, radishes, red onions, cauliflower, artichokes, parsnips, shallots, leeks, sugar snap peas, watercress, olives, etc. You need at least 4 colours per meal.
4)   Count calories.
5)   There are some really cool Apps, which let you scan the packaging and help you determine exactly how many calories you eat and burn e.g. fitnesspal. 6)   Use as little oil, butter as you can, 100 ml of olive oil is 800 calories, 100 g of butter is about 750 calories.
7)   Read the labels and look at the calories, e.g. Muesli, all the various milk types from Rice milk to Quinoa, they are many hidden calories which can be avoided.
8)   Ditch bread for a while, substitute with low calorie crackers.
9)   General rule is the darker the bread the better, e.g. Rye bread.
10) General rule is the darker the lettuce the better.
11) Start the day with protein; I eat two boiled eggs and protein bread just about every day.
12) For snack grab vegetables over fruit. E.g. Carrots, cucumbers, tomatoes, boring I know but look at the calories, low enough that you can eat a lot without feeling guilty. Reach for high taste e.g. Sauerkraut and Gherkins.
13) Talk to yourself, as you feel tempted to grab for something you really don't want to eat.
14) Nuts are out for now.
15) Decide how you feel about dairy products and make a plan. NB: Cheese is super high in calories
16) Add smoked salmon, chicken (not cooked in oil but sautéed with onions in a pan) tuna fish, ham slices to your pile of veggies.
17) Enjoy a baked potato but use a sweet potato not white and add Cottage cheese and a little salt, filling and warming.

18) Look out for false friends: e.g. Dried fruit, 100 g of dried apple is 333 calories. 19) Sit down to eat and take stock of what you are eating.

20) Put everything you intend to eat on your plate and then eat, no adding once you have sat down.

21) Eat, clear up and LEAVE the kitchen.

22) Have a go to solution when you want something sweet, for me this is a Hot Chocolate, the powder mixed with water mix; they can be about 50 calories.

APPENDIX C: CHAPTER TOP TIPS ON ONE PAGE:
1:
GOLD TIP: It is definitely easier to start on a triathlon adventure with a group of friends or a club. Go out and find similar minded friends with whom you can discover triathlon. If you prefer, go to a tri club if you are that kind of person or drag a friend with you to your local club.
SILVER: Be brave talk about your new found interest in triathlon. You will be amazed how many people are already doing Tri and how they want to talk about it, you will learn a lot.
BRONZE: Look up events near you, which you can go and watch or even volunteer at OR better still, sign up and do one, a small one, a short one, tell no one and just go and try it out OR organise your own private one.

2:
GOLD TIP: Consider your rational and irrational motivators. Use the table in Chapter 19 and write them down and develop them over time.
SILVER: On a run, use the alone time to analyse yourself, your strengths and weaknesses.
BRONZE: Consider how you go about your daily tasks. What might by your mantra for life?

3:
GOLD TIP: Keep a record of how much water you are drinking in a day, and how well you are feeling when you are training. Monitor energy levels and general level of enjoyment.
SILVER: Pain can be your friend. Get to know and understand your different types of pain. Some pain you should push through, others pain, definitely not. BRONZE: If you feel seasick in the water, do 6 somersaults in a row every day and eat ginger.

4:
GOLD TIP: Record all your training and at the end of the week add up the distances and hours spent on all disciplines. Specifically, compare intended training session and actual training session. This way you will learn to be flexible in a week's training.
SILVER: Become informed on your anatomy; learn about muscles and fascia, the skeleton and cartilage. Record any aches and pains so you can see if a pattern is developing.
BRONZE: Train with a friend or SMS your training plans frequently to a friend if you can, so that s/he can see when you are over training or pushing an injury too far and

s/he can tell you to stop. Sometimes you need someone else to give you permission to slow down.

5:
GOLD TIP: Always carry an Ibuprofen with you, whether it is a half marathon or an ultra distance triathlon, you never know.
SILVER: Most of us mortals need to build up the distances slowly; most of us cannot pull off a Maria.
BRONZE: Try and run after a long bike session even if it is only 2 km.

6:
GOLD TIP: Use two swim caps, and put your goggles on between the two caps. Do this often as you practice at the pool, to practice how it feels. This prevents cap and goggle loss on the day!
SILVER: A friend sent me good luck wishes, "swim like a fish, run like a hare and bike as if you are wearing the yellow jersey." I kept repeating that all race day. By the way, fish have no arms, it is all core... The tip is to find your race day mantra, be on the look out for it in the last few days before the race. BRONZE: Many professional and experienced athletes like to race at a certain "race weight." See Appendix B for (race) weight loss strategies. According to Rory Coleman of Marathon de Sable fame (look him up, interesting character,) to lose weight, you have to stop eating bread, pasta, rice etc. When he said this to us, we asked, " what about the carbs you need to train?" He replied, "You are wearing them." You have to be wise about this of course. We never really lost serious weight, much to our enormous disappointment.

7:
GOLD: Try this breathing exercise: See how few breaths you can take in a 3-minute period. Professional athletes can get as low as three. Sometimes it forces a type of panic and leads to greedily snatching breaths. This comes close to how I felt in the swim. Practice this and record your improvement. This is easily done in the car, on the train, bus, while waiting for someone. . See: youtube.com/watch?v=S6BGyY7jTX0 or www.yogabasics.com/practice/dirga-pranayama/
SILVER When you swim, swim intelligently, focussed and with precision. Better to swim 1000m of good stroke than 2000 sloppily. This is similar to wasted miles when running.
BRONZE: Read up about what constitutes good swim technique, watch videos and try to emulate the professionals.

8:

GOLD TIP: Engaging a swim teacher is a good idea. S/he will teach you how to swim and train properly so there are no wasted lengths in the pool. This has two benefits. Number one you will not emerge so exhausted from the swim portion and two you will learn to save leg energy, which is crucial for the next part of your triathlon day. A good technique will give you a good rhythm and that will help with stabilizing your heart rate. Crucial is the bilateral breathing, which you really should master especially in the open water situation. Also you will need to learn to sight the buoys.

SILVER: Swimming at the pool can get boring and well into the training schedule it might become a chore. Going with someone helps. We used to split up the 1000m stretches into 100m challenges. I would determine what we did for 4 lengths and then Kirsten would determine the next 4 and so on. This kept our minds working because we always had to come up with a new challenge, no repetition. E.g. just arms with open fingers or fists, sprints, crawl legs and breaststroke arms. Anything we could think of to trick the mind into having a good time.

BRONZE: For sighting practice (which is teaching you to keep going in the right direction,) we would place a float or water bottle at the far end of the pool and look for it every 5 breaths. The smaller the sighting item, the better because it forced us to focus.

9:

GOLD: Learn about the technique of visualisation as a mental tool. Start practicing it on your runs, swims and bike rides.

SILVER: Develop a visualisation library, using the events (marathons, swims etc.) you complete as part of your visualization library. Add certain places from your training repertoire to this library. I often use a 400-metre outdoor athletics track we used to train on in Spain when on my treadmill to push myself through a turbo running session. I picture myself running around this track, passing the pole-vaulters, the high jumpers, the sprinters warming up and the spectator stands. I became so good at this technique that when on a long solo bike ride I could reduce myself to tears visualising myself crossing the IRONMAN finish line! BRONZE: Study the course map before the race and come up with a hydration and nutrition plan.

10:

GOLD TIP: You just never ever know how the day will turn out, but most important, don't push yourself too far, keep going but always be safe.

SILVER: A repeat but I think it is important to recognize the impact of a mantra. Let it flow, breathe, find your mantra even in the toughest of situations. Quoting Gerry Duffy, the total nut who completed ten ultra distance triathlons in ten days, again from his book," Tick Tock Ten," he survived by counting backwards, e.g. 180 to bike, 179, 178 etc., 41 km to run 40 km to run through to 3 km to run 2, 1 and each km he celebrated! It is a book well worth reading.

BRONZE: It doesn't matter if you come in nearly last, finishing is still an awesome achievement. Because as John Bingham said "The miracle is not that I finished, it is that I had the courage to start."

11:

GOLD TIP: If you want something enough it can be yours. Channel your anger and indignation or fear of failure into something positive.

SILVER: Learn from a DNF- Did Not Finish... "That which does not kill us, makes us stronger" - Friedrich Nietzsche

BRONZE: Triathlon is not only an individual sport; it is also very much a team sport. If you include your IRONMAN wherever you did it on your CV, be prepared to explain that it is not simply an individual event.

12:

GOLD TIP: Welcome this new aspect of your personality. Have to say sometimes I fear being boring, talking about kids, school, family, work, etc., this is at least a new dimension. (I know I can get boring about triathlete/sport/nutrition too!) SILVER: Try and incorporate your training into your family life. I would often train in a nearby park as Tobias warmed up for and played the first half of his basketball match and then watch the second half.

BRONZE: Think about fund-raising for a charity.

13:

GOLD TIP: Work on a mental strategy, by now you should understand your mental strengths and weaknesses. Talk to yourself. Examine your fears now in you mind. Let your mind wander through these fears and dig into them. Better to do this now than on race day. Scan your visualisation library; keep it up to date and ready for the challenge ahead. Remind yourself what gives you positive energy on race day. For me I enjoy interacting with the crowd. People might cheer and shout, "keep going Tiffany," I love that encouragement, I will nearly always respond.

SILVER: Follow your tapering plan to the letter; do not overdo anything. As scary as that feels, it is much more beneficial at this stage to stay lying on the couch, feet up, than to go for a run or bike or swim.

BRONZE: Read chapter 26 to understand that being pretty nervous is very much part of this journey.

14:

GOLD: Revel, I mean revel in your achievement; you are AWESOME.
SILVER: Write an account of your day so that when you feel down you can read about how wonderful you were/are.
BRONZE: Take some time off and keep revelling.

15:
GOLD TIP: Definitely get the tattoo. If I were to do it again, I would place it on my left calf half way up my leg so it could be seen by runners behind me. No one sees it at the side!
SILVER: Give your bike ride trail a personality. Name various spots or stretches. Love them and hate them.
BRONZE: Take one section of this ride and time how long it takes to do this stretch. Keep a record and see your times improve.

16:
GOLD TIP: Look at the course map and select the best vantage point for your spectators in advance, estimate where and when you will be at certain spots, mark them on the course map, that way they will enjoy the day and want to come to support you again.
SILVER: Take good care of your supporters; make sure they have water and snacks and a camera. Often races have a tracking App, download this for them, enter your race number and get them prepared.
BRONZE: Take a B event like Buitrago and make a social event out of it. The Buitrago half was an excellent training event but was also so much fun.

17:
GOLD TIP: Be prepared for the mental battle. It is fierce and draining, even if you are not menopausal, not moving house or are miles from the venue.
SILVER: On the other hand you have to enjoy the run up to an event such as this. You are fit, probably more or less injury-free, about to embark on a day in your life that you will remember forever. So embrace all the sensations, record them if you are a diarist, or take photos.
BRONZE: Use a checklist as you pack each bag and load stuff into the car.

18:
GOLD TIP: Plan your finisher photo; leave about 2 seconds between you and the person ahead of you in order to get a clear finisher photo with just you on it. In Zürich the guy right in front of me hogged the photo, by Roth, I had learned my lesson, the

camera caught just me on the image. You don't want to share that frame with anyone else.
SILVER: Turbo run and turbo bike as frequently as you can handle it.
BRONZE: It is much, much easier to go to a triathlon event by car than by plane.

19:
GOLD: New dreams, new goals, new people, new experiences AND new equipment...
SILVER: If you still need to participate in a triathlon, there are always triathlon relay teams.
BRONZE: Be grateful it is nothing more serious.

Please feel free to contact me on female_ironman@hotmail.com I would love to hear from you. Please tell me about your own triathlon, ultra running and or other (sporting) achievements.

I sincerely hope you enjoyed reading this book as much as I enjoyed writing it. Look out for my next title, which is still very much in the "warm-up" stage. Working title, "All I ever wanted was a six pack." It will be something about ultra marathons and trail running, and strong women of course.

Huge thanks........

I would like to thank my fabulous family for supporting me in my adventures. They have always offered enormous encouragement not only for my training and events but also for my latest project of endurance, this book. Particularly, I would like to thank my daughters, Sacha, Tatjana and Natasja for painstakingly reading through my multiple drafts, offering insightful suggestions and making keen observations always delivered tactfully and sensitively!

I would also like to thank Barbara (check her out on boostingnow.com) who read my ugly first draft and helped me shape the text and ideas into a proper book with structure. Secondly, I would like to thank Tiffany, (my friend,) who picked through every sentence with enormous patience, corrected the grammar and added thousands of commas. Let me know when I can baby-sit your kids, clean your kitchen or do your ironing in return for the great favour you both extended to me. Finally a thank you goes out to Thomas who did the artwork for the book cover. The first impression was the last element of the book to be completed, I owe you one Thomas, merci.

References:

[2] www.runnersworld.com/health/running-empty

[3] http://www.bengreenfieldfitness.com/2009/05/why/

[4] (https://www.quora.com/What-percentage-of-the-worlds-population-has-completed-an-Ironman-Triathlon

[5] http://1.bp.blogspot.com/-cEGzabXqGrw/UBluDEEGU-I/AAAAAAAAS1M/OI31YrY9DAY/s1600/Ironman+Finishers+as+Percent+of+Gender+by+Continent+and+Event+by+Raymond+Britt.png

[6] http://www.elle.com/beauty/health-fitness/advice/a14560/the-women-of-ironman

[7] https://www.collinsdictionary.com/dictionary/english/aquaphobia

[8] http://www.denverpost.com/2013/07/08/triathlons-other-endurance-races-higher-death-risk-for-middle-aged/

[9] http://www.bloomberg.com/news/articles/2013-06-20/men-over-40-should-think-twice-before-running-triathlons

[10] http://www.point2lapointe.com

[11] http://www.drivingtesttips.biz/motorway-road-signs.html#prettyPhoto/9/

[12] www.thetrihub.com

[13] : http://www.ironman.com/triathlon-news/articles/2013/07/secrets-of-the-course-ironman-switzerland.aspx#ixzz4Yvgo7wEC

[14] http://www.ironman.com/triathlon/events/emea/ironman/Switzerland/athletes/results.aspx#ixzz31Ul03WKN

[15] https://upload.wikimedia.org/wikipedia/commons/2/2e/Clavicle_-_animation.gif

[16] http://dailyquotes.co/12-things-successful-people-do-differently/

[17] http://bicycles.stackexchange.com/questions/244/terminology-index-a-list-of-bike-part-names-and-cycling-concepts

[18] http://www.take-ten.com/daily-positive-quotes/its-amazing-how-far-you-can-go-just-because-someone-believed-in-you-positive-thought-of-the-day-by-taketen

Made in the USA
Columbia, SC
19 July 2019